The Pink Salt Trick Diet for Weight Loss

> Harness the Power of Himalayan Pink Salt for Natural Weight Loss, Detox, and Metabolism Boosting Recipes. Includes a 30-Day Meal Plan with Recipes.

Denise J. Maclennan

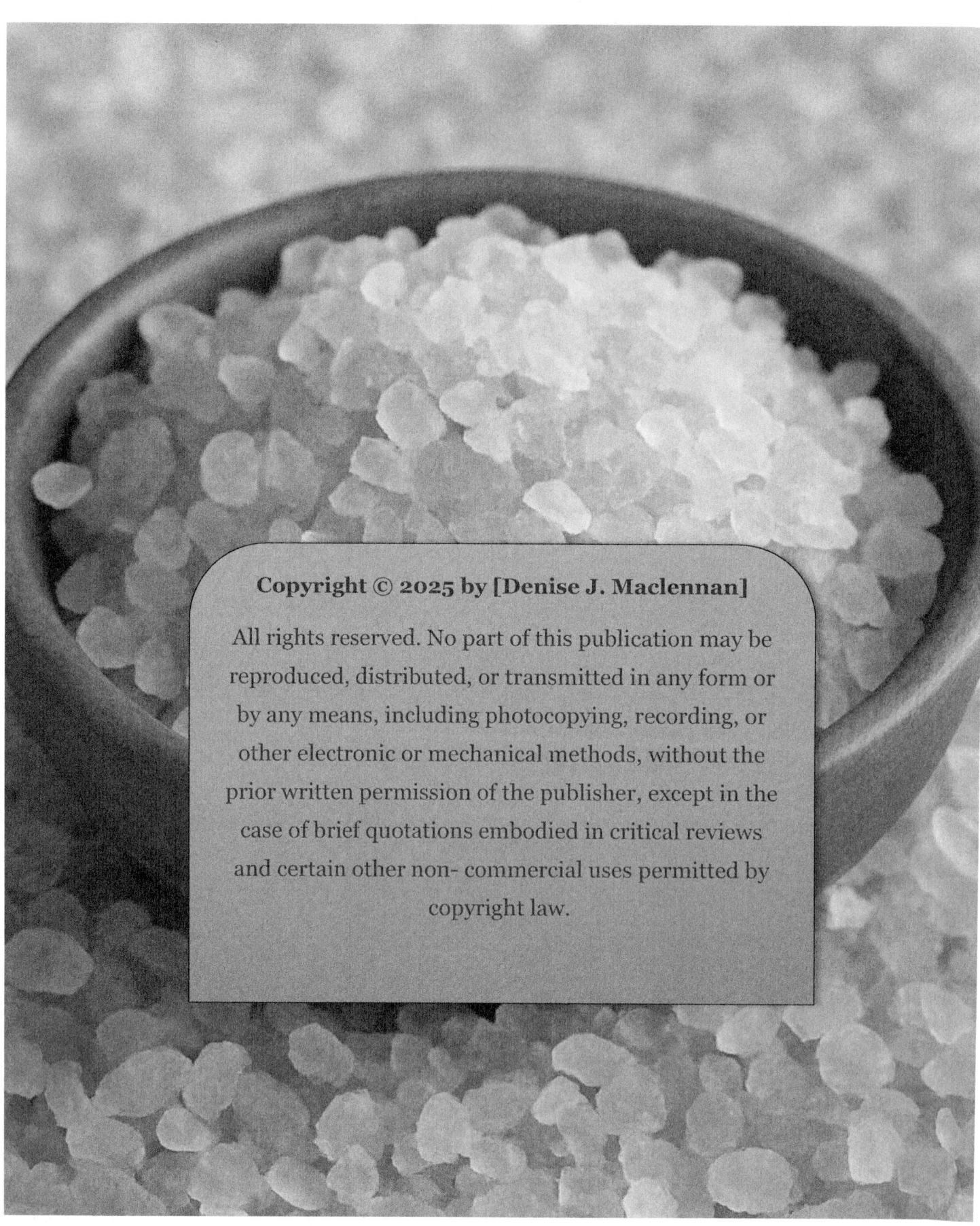

Copyright © 2025 by [Denise J. Maclennan]

All rights reserved. No part of this publication may be reproduced, distributed, or transmitted in any form or by any means, including photocopying, recording, or other electronic or mechanical methods, without the prior written permission of the publisher, except in the case of brief quotations embodied in critical reviews and certain other non- commercial uses permitted by copyright law.

Table of Contents

Introduction 7
    Why This Book Matters 9
    My Personal Journey with the Pink Salt Trick....... 9
    What You'll Gain from This Book...................... 10
    How to Use This Book..................................... 11

Chapter 1: Understanding The Pink Salt Trick Diet 13
    What is the "Pink Salt Trick"? 13
    Why Himalayan Pink Salt? 14
        Origin and Composition............................ 15
        Mineral Content and Benefits..................... 17
        Pink Salt vs. Table Salt............................... 19
    How It Works for Weight Loss 21
        Detoxification Mechanism.......................... 23
        Appetite Control & Cravings Reduction 24
        Balancing Electrolytes & Boosting Metabolism 26
    Scientific Insights and Evidence....................... 27
    Misconceptions & Cautions 29
    How Much Pink Salt is Safe to Consume? 31
    The Pink Salt Morning Flush Explained 33

Chapter 2: Getting Started with the Pink Salt Lifestyle 35
    Preparing Your Pantry 35
    Recommended Kitchen Tools........................... 37
    Shopping List for the First Week...................... 38
    Reading Food Labels & Sodium Awareness........ 40
    Portion Sizes & Serving Tips 41
    Hydration and the Role of Water...................... 43
    Supplements & Synergistic Superfoods 44
    Exercise and Mindful Eating Pairings 45

Chapter 3: Breakfast Recipes 48
    Pink Salt Morning Detox Water........................ 49
    Avocado Toast with Pink Salt & Chili Flakes....... 49
    Pink Salt Veggie Omelette 50
    Greek Yogurt Parfait with Pink Salted Granola... 50
    Chia Pudding with Pink Salted Mango 51
    Almond Butter Pink Salt Smoothie.................... 51
    Protein Pancakes with Pink Salted Berries......... 52
    Overnight Oats with Himalayan Sea Salt & Figs . 52
    Breakfast Quinoa Bowl with Banana and Pink Salt 53
    Tofu Scramble with Pink Salt........................... 53
    Cinnamon-Spiced Apple Bake with Pink Salt...... 54
    Blueberry Protein Shake with Pink Salt.............. 54
    Pink Salt & Turmeric Coconut Milk 55
    Gluten-Free Breakfast Muffins with a Pink Salt Twist... 55
    Zucchini Hash with Poached Egg and Pink Salt.. 56

Chapter 4: Lunch Recipes 57
    Grilled Chicken Salad with Pink Salt Citrus Dressing 58
    Pink Salt Tuna Lettuce Wraps........................... 58
    Roasted Veggie & Quinoa Bowl with Pink Salt.... 59

Chickpea Salad with Cucumber, Dill & Pink Salt .59
Zesty Pink Salt Shrimp Stir-Fry 60
Lentil Soup with Pink Salt and Thyme 60
Pink Salted Kale and Avocado Rice Bowl 61
Baked Falafel with Pink Salt & Tahini Sauce 61
Asian Slaw with Pink Salt Sesame Dressing 62
Pink Salt Marinated Grilled Tofu Bowl 62
Mushroom and Pink Salt Risotto 63
Turmeric Chicken and Pink Salt Couscous 63
Stuffed Bell Peppers with Pink Salt Quinoa Mix .64

Chapter 5: Dinner Recipes 65
Lemon Garlic Salmon with Pink Salt 66
Pink Salt Chicken Stir-Fry with Veggies 66
Vegan Cauliflower & Chickpea Curry 67
Baked Pink Salted Cod with Citrus Zest 67
Roasted Turkey Meatballs with Pink Salt 68
Stir-Fried Tofu and Broccoli in Pink Salt Sauce . 68
Grilled Eggplant with Pink Salt Herb Drizzle 69
Sautéed Spinach & Mushrooms with Pink Salt.... 69
Zucchini Noodles with Pink Salt Tomato Sauce ..70
Herbed Basmati Rice with Pink Salt 70
Pink Salt Chili Lime Chicken Skewers 71
Stuffed Zucchini Boats with Pink Salt 71
Moroccan Chickpea Stew with Pink Salt 72
Thai-Inspired Pink Salt Coconut Soup 72
Teriyaki Glazed Tempeh with Pink Salt 73

Chapter 6: Snacks, Smoothies & Light Bites 74
Pink Salt Dark Chocolate Almond Bites 75
Pink Salt Sweet Potato Chips 75
Avocado Salsa with Pink Salt 76
Pink Salt Edamame Pods 76
Spiced Carrot Hummus with Pink Salt 77
Pink Salt Nut & Seed Trail Mix 77
Detox Smoothie with Cucumber, Mint & Pink Salt 78
Pink Salt Watermelon & Mint Salad 78
Protein Bars with Pink Salt & Cranberries 79
Spicy Pink Salt Roasted Chickpeas 79
Strawberry Coconut Shake with Pink Salt 80
Almond-Coconut Balls with a Pink Salt Twist.....80
Green Smoothie with Lemon & Pink Salt 81
Roasted Seaweed Snack with Pink Salt 81
Frozen Banana Bites with Pink Salt & Cocoa 82

Chapter 7: The 30-Day Pink Salt Trick Meal Plan 83
How to Follow the 30-Day Plan 83
🍽 Calorie Guidance for Weight Loss 84
🍽 Customization Tips (Vegetarian, Vegan, Gluten-Free) 86
Weekly Shopping Lists 88
Weekly Prep Instructions 92
▶ Week 1: Detox & Flush 95
▶ Week 2: Fat Burn & Stabilize 96
▶ Week 3: Metabolism Boost 97
▶ Week 4: Tone & Sustain 98

Chapter 8: Expert Tips for Long-Term Success 99
Avoiding Plateaus: When Progress Slows........... 99

Adapting the Pink Salt Trick After 30 Days 101

Making It a Lifestyle, Not a Phase 103

Meal Prepping for Busy Weeks 106

Pink Salt in Restaurant Eating 108

Staying Motivated & Measuring Progress 111

Chapter 9: Frequently Asked Questions 114

Can I use pink salt if I have high blood pressure? 114

Will I lose weight just by adding pink salt? 115

What are signs of overconsumption? 116

Can I combine this with intermittent fasting? ... 118

What if I miss a day of the trick? 119

Chapter 10: Measurement Conversions & Nutritional Guidelines 122

Metric/Imperial Conversion Charts 122

Portion Size Guide 124

Understanding Macronutrients 126

Conclusion 129

Free Gift 130

🙏 **Acknowledgements 131**

Recipe Index 132

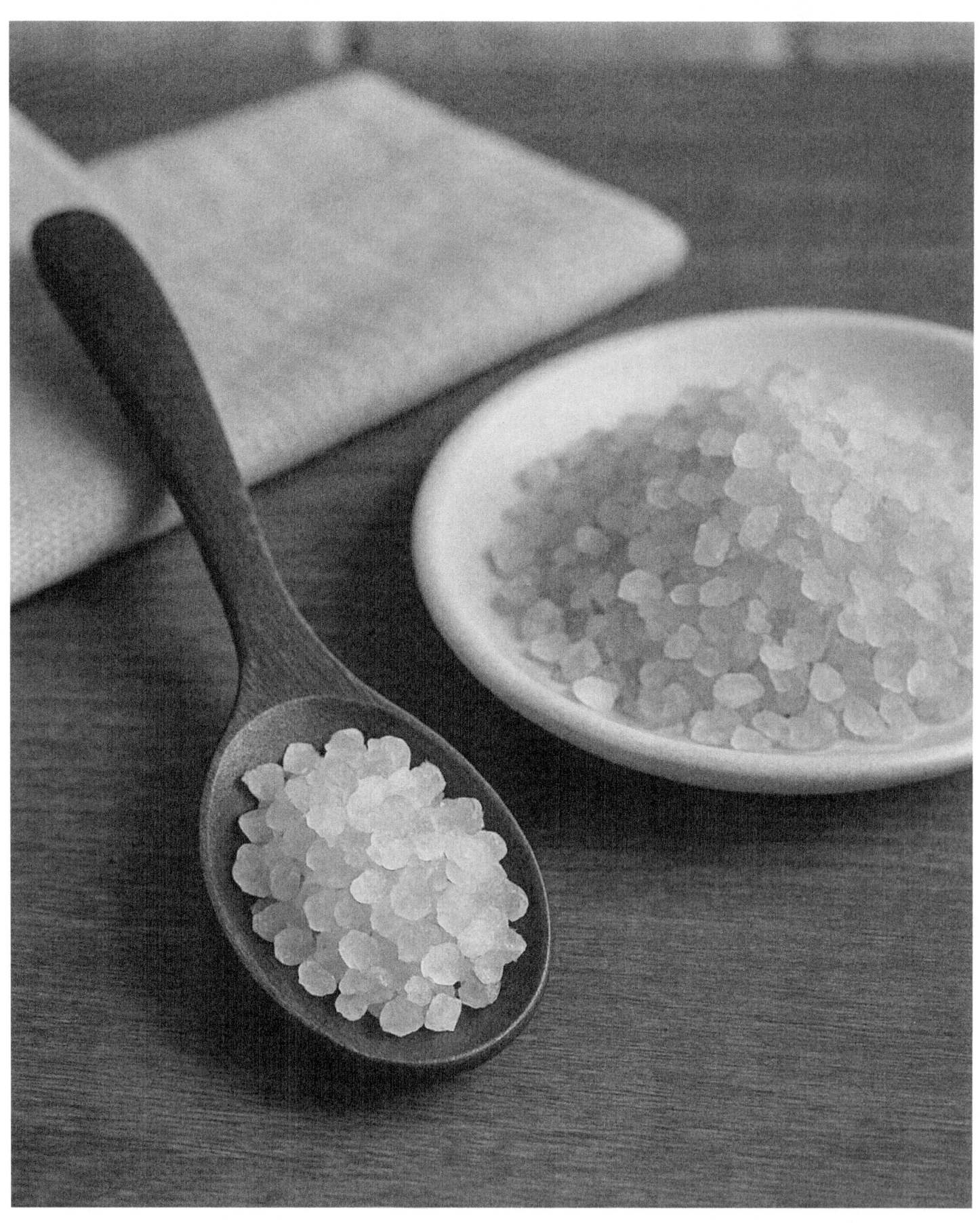

INTRODUCTION

Welcome to ***The Pink Salt Trick Diet for Weight Loss***—your gateway to a natural, sustainable, and nourishing approach to health and wellness.

In a world filled with diet fads, chemical detoxes, and overwhelming meal restrictions, the simplicity and effectiveness of Himalayan pink salt has quietly emerged as a game-changer. This book isn't about deprivation or chasing rapid results. It's about tapping into the unique mineral power of pink salt to support your body's natural metabolism, reduce cravings, and gently detoxify—without sacrificing flavor or enjoyment.

You might be wondering: *How can something as simple as salt help with weight loss?*

That's the heart of what we're exploring here. The **"Pink Salt Trick"** refers to a specific method of incorporating high-quality Himalayan pink salt into your daily routine—in precise, purposeful ways—to help:

- Kickstart digestion and fat burning,
- Replenish essential minerals,
- Regulate water retention,
- And reduce unhealthy cravings for processed foods.

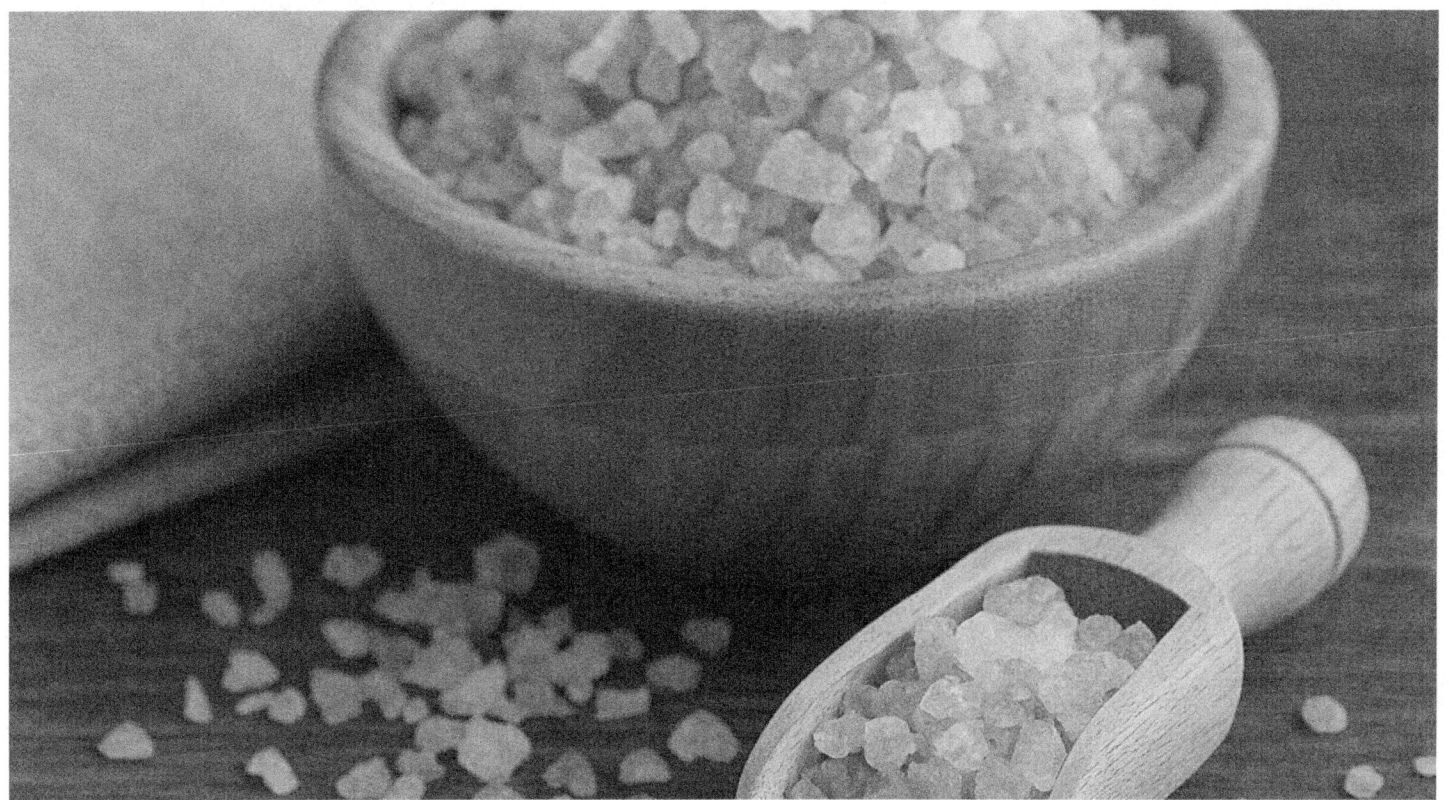

Why This Book Was Written

Like many others, I was once stuck in a cycle of constant dieting, fatigue, and frustration. My discovery of the Pink Salt Trick didn't happen overnight—it came after researching natural wellness practices, consulting nutritionists, and experimenting in my own kitchen. The results were undeniable: steady weight loss, boosted energy, better sleep, and an overall lighter, more vibrant feeling in my body.

This book is the product of that journey—fueled by personal transformation and backed by science. And now, it's your turn.

What You'll Discover

This is more than a recipe collection. It's a complete lifestyle guide built around a simple yet effective strategy. Inside, you'll find:

- A crystal-clear explanation of how the Pink Salt Trick works
- 60 nutrient-packed, delicious recipes enhanced with pink salt
- A full 30-day meal plan to take the guesswork out of your journey
- Expert tips for staying on track and avoiding common pitfalls
- Guidance on how to make this a permanent, enjoyable lifestyle

Whether you're new to healthy eating or already on your wellness path, this book is designed to meet you where you are—with flexibility, support, and inspiration.

A Gentle Word Before You Begin

This is not a magic solution—but it is a powerful tool. When paired with intentional eating, hydration, and self-care, the Pink Salt Trick can unlock new levels of wellness that feel sustainable and natural. Think of it as a reset—not just for your body, but for your relationship with food.

So grab your pink salt, tie on your apron, and let's embark on a flavorful, empowering journey toward the best version of you—one mindful, mineral-rich meal at a time.

Let's begin.

Why This Book Matters

In an era where health advice often feels contradictory, overcomplicated, or out of reach, The Pink Salt Trick Diet for Weight Loss offers something rare: clarity, simplicity, and science-backed effectiveness.

This book matters because it reintroduces readers to something ancient yet often overlooked—**Himalayan pink salt**—and teaches you how to use it not just as seasoning, but as a powerful wellness ally.

Here's why this book could change your wellness journey:

- **It Demystifies Natural Weight Loss:** Instead of relying on extreme calorie restriction or costly supplements, this book shows you how natural mineral balance—starting with pink salt—can gently stimulate weight loss, balance hormones, and enhance energy.
- **It Puts the Power Back in Your Hands:** No fad diets. No unrealistic promises. Just real food, real strategies, and real transformation—centered around your lifestyle, your preferences, and your goals.
- **It's Grounded in Purpose, Not Gimmicks:** Every recipe and recommendation in this book has been intentionally designed to support your metabolism, reduce bloating, and help you feel lighter, clearer, and more in control—without sacrificing enjoyment.
- **It Helps You Reset Without Starving:** Many people associate detoxing with deprivation. This book takes a different approach—offering flavorful, satisfying meals that nourish your body while helping it naturally detox and re-balance.
- **It Works With Your Body, Not Against It:** Himalayan pink salt, when used correctly, helps regulate hydration, supports adrenal function, and improves nutrient absorption. It's not just about cutting calories—it's about giving your body what it truly needs to thrive.

This book matters because your health matters—and sustainable, joyful wellness shouldn't feel like a mystery or a luxury.

If you've ever felt frustrated, stuck, or discouraged by confusing health advice or diets that left you drained, this book offers a fresh, empowering alternative.

Let's simplify, reset, and begin anew—with purpose, knowledge, and a pinch of pink salt.

My Personal Journey with the Pink Salt Trick

Before this book was a reality, it began as a deeply personal journey.

Like many, I struggled with weight that seemed to creep up year after year. I wasn't overeating junk food or skipping workouts—but I felt **bloated, tired, and frustrated.** Every "diet" I tried left me either starving or stressed, and worst of all, nothing seemed to last. I began to question whether long-term weight loss was even possible without extreme measures.

That all changed the day I stumbled upon something so simple, it almost sounded too good to be true: **a pink mineral salt from the Himalayas.**

I had heard whispers of people using Himalayan pink salt in water first thing in the morning for energy, digestion, even weight loss. Skeptical but curious, I began experimenting—slowly and mindfully—integrating this salt into my daily routine.

The results were subtle at first, but powerful.

- **I woke up less bloated.**
- **My cravings dropped dramatically.**
- **My digestion improved.**
- **I felt lighter—physically and mentally.**

What started as a daily pink salt drink quickly became a foundation for deeper change. I adjusted my meals, paired ingredients more mindfully, and began creating flavorful recipes that supported my goals without sacrificing enjoyment.

Over a few months, I lost weight naturally, my skin looked clearer, my sleep improved, and I no longer dreaded stepping on the scale. But more importantly, I finally felt in control of my health—without extremes, without shame, and without guesswork.

That experience is what inspired this book.

I realized that I wasn't alone. So many others are searching for balance—a way to nourish their body, lose weight, and feel good again without being overwhelmed by conflicting advice.

This book is the guide I wish I had when I started.

It's a toolkit, a collection of everything I've learned—from how to use pink salt safely and effectively, to delicious recipes that turn clean eating into something exciting and deeply satisfying.

It's not magic. It's not a miracle cure. But it is a proven, natural method that supports your body's ability to heal, shed excess weight, and thrive.

And I'm honored to share it with you.

Let this be the start of your journey—because if it worked for me, it can work for you too.

With encouragement,

What You'll Gain from This Book

This isn't just another diet book—it's your **practical blueprint** for sustainable weight loss, natural detox, and joyful eating, all built around one simple yet powerful tool: **Himalayan pink salt.**

By the time you finish this book, you'll have more than just knowledge—you'll have a clear plan, tools that work, and recipes that inspire. Whether you're beginning your wellness journey or looking to reset your habits, this book will meet you where you are—and move you forward.

Here's exactly what you'll gain:

🔍 A Clear Understanding of the "Pink Salt Trick"

- What it is, how it works, and why it's so effective for weight loss and detox
- How pink salt differs from regular salt—and why quality matters
- How to use the trick daily, safely, and effectively

🧠 Science-Backed Knowledge

- The role of trace minerals in metabolism, hydration, digestion, and fat burn
- Insights into how pink salt can support adrenal health, reduce sugar cravings, and balance your body

🍱 60 Delicious, Metabolism-Boosting Recipes

- Breakfasts, lunches, dinners, snacks, smoothies, and light bites—all featuring pink salt in balanced, flavorful ways
- Meals designed to support your energy, reduce inflammation, and keep you full without overeating

📅 A 30-Day Guided Meal Plan

- No guesswork—just a structured plan that aligns meals, hydration, and salt timing to maximize results
- Week-by-week themes to help your body detox, stabilize, burn fat, and sustain energy

💪 Practical Lifestyle Tools

- How to prep your pantry and kitchen
- Shopping guides and batch cooking tips
- Hydration and salt balance strategies
- Tips for dining out, social events, and busy weeks

💡 Confidence & Control

- Know how to listen to your body and adjust your approach
- Learn how to turn weight loss from a painful struggle into a mindful practice
- Feel empowered with real tools—not marketing gimmicks or temporary fixes

This book isn't here to overwhelm you—it's here to equip you. You'll walk away with a better relationship with food, more awareness of your body, and the confidence to take control of your health using one of nature's simplest but most powerful gifts.

Your journey doesn't have to be hard.

It just has to begin—with the right guidance.

How to Use This Book

This book is designed to be your personal roadmap to weight loss, detox, and improved vitality using the power of Himalayan pink salt. Whether you're just starting your wellness journey or seeking a new approach that actually fits your lifestyle, this book is laid out to guide you step by step—without confusion or overwhelm.

Here's how to make the most of it:

🔑 Start with the Foundation (Chapters 1–2)

Before diving into recipes, take time to read the first two chapters. These explain the science, logic, and health principles behind the Pink Salt Trick:

- Learn how and why it works
- Understand the right way to use pink salt (and how much is safe)
- Get clarity on what to expect, especially in the first week

This foundation ensures you're not just following blindly—you're making informed choices that empower you long-term.

🍽 Explore the 60 Recipes (Chapters 3–6)

Each recipe has been crafted to balance nutrition, flavor, and function. Feel free to:

- Follow the meal plan exactly OR mix and match based on your preferences

- Substitute proteins or vegetables based on your dietary needs
- Batch cook or meal prep based on your schedule

Use the recipe sections like a menu—something you'll come back to again and again.

1️⃣ Follow the 30-Day Meal Plan (Chapter 7)

Once you've grasped the basics, move to the 30-day plan. It's broken into 4 weekly phases, each with:

- A specific focus (detox, fat burn, metabolism boost, maintenance)
- Pre-planned meals and hydration tips
- A shopping list and light prep guide to save time

This structure removes the guesswork and helps you build momentum right away.

📇 Refer to the Lifestyle & Tips Section (Chapters 8–10)

These chapters are your long-term support system. Inside, you'll find:

- Success tips and real-life guidance
- Frequently asked questions (with science-backed answers)
- Measurement conversions, serving suggestions, and nutrition advice

These are the tools to help you turn results into a sustainable lifestyle.

✅ Customize Your Experience

This is your journey. Adapt the plan to:

- Accommodate vegetarian, gluten-free, or dairy-free diets
- Fit around work, travel, or family commitments
- Progress at a pace that feels right for your body

The Pink Salt Trick isn't one-size-fits-all—it's flexible, realistic, and built to evolve with you.

Final Tip: Don't Strive for Perfection—Strive for Consistency.

If you miss a day, feel tired, or eat something off-plan, don't stress. Just return to the process and keep going. This book isn't about doing everything right—it's about doing what's right for you.

Now, let's begin your transformation—one mineral-rich, healing meal at a time.

CHAPTER 1: UNDERSTANDING THE PINK SALT TRICK DIET

What is the "Pink Salt Trick"?

At the heart of this book lies a deceptively simple yet profoundly effective method for jumpstarting natural weight loss, improving digestion, and restoring mineral balance: **the Pink Salt Trick.**

But what exactly is it?

🧂 **The "Pink Salt Trick" is the practice of consuming a small, measured amount of Himalayan pink salt dissolved in warm water—typically first thing in the morning—on an empty stomach.**

This practice is often referred to as a **"pink salt flush"** or **mineral tonic,** and when paired with a clean, supportive diet (as provided in this book), it can help:

- 🔥 Stimulate metabolism
- 🚽 Support healthy elimination and detoxification
- 💧 Rebalance hydration and electrolyte levels
- 😋 Reduce cravings and stabilize mood
- 🧘 Promote a feeling of fullness and calm

Why Does This Simple Trick Work?

Unlike regular table salt, which is heavily processed and stripped of nutrients, Himalayan pink salt is a natural, unrefined salt rich in over 80 trace minerals, including:

- Magnesium
- Potassium
- Calcium
- Iron
- Zinc

These minerals are critical for metabolic health, adrenal function, nerve signaling, and fluid balance—all of which influence weight regulation and energy levels.

When consumed in a measured dose, pink salt:

- Encourages gentle detox through the bowels
- Enhances nutrient absorption in the gut
- Signals satiety and reduces sugar cravings
- Replenishes lost minerals—especially important if you're stressed or exercising

The Pink Salt Trick in Practice

The basic method is simple:

1. Mix ¼ to ½ teaspoon of Himalayan pink salt in 8–12 ounces of warm water

2. Drink it immediately upon waking, before any food or coffee

3. Wait about 30 minutes before eating breakfast

4. Follow up with plenty of clean water throughout the day

This routine kickstarts your system like a natural detox switch—without chemicals, pills, or extreme fasting.

📝 **Important:** The "trick" isn't just the salt—it's the timing, hydration, and consistency paired with the right nutrition that makes this method truly effective.

What It's Not:

✘ Not a magic weight loss potion

✘ Not a replacement for proper nutrition

✘ Not a laxative or extreme cleanse

It's a gentle, nourishing tool to help your body work the way it's meant to—by supporting your internal systems with essential minerals and smart habits.

A Word on Safety

When done properly and in moderation, the Pink Salt Trick is safe for most healthy adults. However, if you have hypertension, kidney issues, or are on sodium-restricted diets, consult your physician before beginning.

Why Himalayan Pink Salt?

If you've ever wondered what makes Himalayan pink salt so special—and why it's at the core of this diet—you're not alone. In a world filled with dozens of salt options, it's important to understand why this particular salt stands out.

Himalayan pink salt isn't just a pretty kitchen trend—it's one of the purest and most mineral-rich salts available on Earth. Mined from the ancient salt beds of the Himalayan Mountains, this pink-hued crystal has remained untouched by pollutants, toxins, and modern processing—making it a natural powerhouse for health and wellness.

⛰️ A Salt Formed by Time and Nature

Over 250 million years ago, prehistoric oceans dried up, leaving behind vast salt deposits deep beneath the earth's surface in what is now Pakistan. These salt veins, shielded from contamination, became compressed under intense geological pressure—preserving their original mineral content.

When you consume Himalayan pink salt, you're tapping into an ancient, natural mineral source formed long before industrial pollution existed.

🔬 What's Inside: The Mineral Breakdown

Unlike refined table salt—which is chemically bleached, stripped of minerals, and often laced with anti-caking agents—Himalayan pink salt contains over 80 essential trace minerals, including:

- **Magnesium** – Calms nerves, reduces water retention, and supports metabolism
- **Potassium** – Helps regulate fluid balance and blood pressure
- **Calcium** – Aids in bone strength and muscle function
- **Iron** – Supports oxygen transport and energy production
- **Zinc** – Boosts immunity and healing
- **Iodine (natural)** – Supports thyroid health (in smaller amounts than iodized salt)

These minerals give Himalayan pink salt its distinct pink hue and its unique ability to help the body detoxify, hydrate, and energize naturally.

💧 Salt That Supports—Not Sabotages—Your Health

When used correctly and in moderation, Himalayan pink salt does far more than just season your food:

- It balances your body's pH, helping reduce inflammation
- It stimulates digestive enzymes, enhancing nutrient absorption
- It supports adrenal function, crucial for managing stress and metabolism
- It helps the body retain the right kind of hydration, avoiding bloating and fatigue
- It works as a gentle detoxifier, drawing out toxins when consumed with water

Unlike conventional salt, which can spike blood pressure and cause water retention when overused, pink salt—thanks to its mineral composition—helps regulate these functions rather than disrupt them.

🌿 A Natural Ally for Weight Loss and Wellness

So why is Himalayan pink salt such a perfect partner for your weight loss journey?

Because it helps address the root causes of weight gain:

- Mineral deficiencies
- Water imbalance
- Cravings and blood sugar swings
- Sluggish digestion and low energy

When you restore balance from the inside out, weight loss becomes natural, not forced. That's why the Pink Salt Trick works so well—it doesn't fight your body. It nourishes it.

Origin and Composition

To truly appreciate the power of Himalayan pink salt, we must begin where it all started—deep within the Earth's crust, in the shadow of the Himalayan Mountains.

This unique salt isn't made in a lab. It wasn't artificially enriched or bleached. It is a naturally formed crystal, harvested from ancient sea beds that existed over 250 million years ago, long before environmental toxins and industrial pollution ever existed.

🌍 Where Does It Come From?

Himalayan pink salt is mined primarily from the **Khewra Salt Mine** in Pakistan, one of the oldest and largest salt mines in the world. Situated at the base of the Himalayas, this underground treasure trove contains vast reserves of salt that have been compressed and preserved under layers of volcanic rock and sediment over millennia.

These ancient salt deposits were formed from the evaporation of prehistoric oceans, then sealed away by tectonic activity, protecting them from environmental exposure. As a result, this salt is remarkably pure and rich in trace elements.

🌿 *Think of it as a mineral time capsule—unrefined, unprocessed, and incredibly potent.*

🧂 What Is It Made Of?

At its core, Himalayan pink salt is composed of:

- **Sodium chloride (NaCl)** – approximately 84–98%, similar to table salt

But what makes it radically different is the 16+% of trace minerals that remain intact.

These include:

- **Magnesium** – supports muscle and nerve function, reduces fatigue
- **Potassium** – helps regulate fluid balance and blood pressure
- **Calcium** – promotes bone and heart hea
- **Iron** – improves energy and oxygen transport, contributes to the salt's pink color
- **Zinc** – aids immunity and metabolism
- **Phosphorus, selenium, copper, manganese,** and others—each playing a role in metabolic and cellular function

In total, over 80 naturally occurring minerals have been identified in high-quality Himalayan salt, giving it both its distinctive pink to deep red color and its earthy, slightly sweet flavor profile.

🏛 Crystalline Structure Matters

Another key feature of Himalayan salt is its intact crystalline structure, formed under immense pressure and heat. This structure:

- Makes the minerals more bioavailable (easier for the body to absorb)
- Contributes to its unique taste and energy-storing potential
- Allows it to be used therapeutically—for example, in baths, lamps, and salt inhalers

Unlike commercial salts that are heated at high temperatures and stripped of nutrients, pink salt's natural crystal matrix remains whole—preserving its full mineral spectrum.

🧂 Why This Matters for Your Health

Your body relies on trace minerals for hundreds of physiological functions:

- Regulating hormones and metabolism
- Facilitating digestion and nutrient uptake
- Managing water retention and electrolyte balance
- Supporting adrenal and thyroid function
- Controlling inflammation and cellular repair

The problem is, modern diets—especially processed foods—are deficient in these minerals. Even many "healthy" diets don't replenish them effectively.

That's where the origin and composition of Himalayan pink salt become powerful: by using a clean, mineral-dense salt daily, you're giving your body essential tools it needs to function optimally—naturally.

Mineral Content and Benefits

Himalayan pink salt isn't just about flavor—it's about function.

What sets it apart from regular salt is its impressive mineral profile. Containing over 80 trace minerals, Himalayan pink salt nourishes your body at a cellular level, offering a host of metabolic, digestive, and detoxifying benefits that directly support weight loss and whole-body wellness.

Let's break down the key minerals and what they do for your body:

🧂 Key Minerals in Himalayan Pink Salt

Mineral	Role in the Body	Weight Loss Benefit
Sodium (Na)	Regulates fluid balance, blood pressure, and nerve impulses	Helps prevent dehydration and supports adrenal function during fat metabolism
Potassium (K)	Supports heart health, fluid balance, and muscle contraction	Balances sodium, reduces bloating, and supports muscle tone
Magnesium (Mg)	Calms nerves, supports sleep, muscle recovery, and blood sugar regulation	Reduces stress-related cravings and promotes fat-burning sleep cycles
Calcium (Ca)	Essential for bone health, muscle function, and hormone signaling	Aids in fat breakdown and stabilizes hunger hormones
Iron (Fe)	Facilitates oxygen transport and energy production	Boosts stamina for physical activity and supports a healthy metabolism
Zinc (Zn)	Supports immunity, hormone balance, and cellular repair	Helps regulate insulin and appetite, improving fat metabolism
Iodine (trace amounts)	Supports thyroid function	Helps regulate metabolism and body temperature
Selenium, Copper, Manganese, and others	Antioxidant defense, enzyme activation, metabolic balance	Reduce inflammation, support detox pathways, and protect cells during fat loss

💡 How These Minerals Boost Health and Weight Loss

1. Electrolyte Balance

Many people struggle with fatigue, water retention, and poor digestion during weight loss. That's often due to an imbalance in electrolytes—especially sodium, potassium, and magnesium. Pink salt restores this balance gently and naturally, reducing bloating and improving hydration without the need for sugary sports drinks.

2. Craving Control

Mineral deficiencies often trigger unexplained cravings for salty or sweet snacks. By restoring your mineral levels with pink salt, your body becomes satisfied more easily, helping reduce compulsive eating and sugar crashes.

3. Improved Digestion

Minerals in pink salt stimulate the production of digestive enzymes and stomach acid, enhancing nutrient absorption and reducing gas, bloating, and sluggish metabolism after meals.

4. Support for Adrenal and Thyroid Health

The adrenal glands and thyroid are central to weight regulation. Pink salt's sodium, magnesium, and trace iodine help support hormonal balance, especially during stress, which is a common trigger for weight gain.

5. Natural Detoxification

Minerals like magnesium, calcium, and selenium help the liver and kidneys flush out toxins efficiently. A properly mineralized body is more efficient at burning fat, because it doesn't need to hold onto excess water or waste for safety.

🧪 Real Results from Real Minerals

Unlike supplements that are often isolated and synthetic, the minerals in pink salt come in whole-food form, allowing your body to absorb them in a balanced, bioavailable way.

💭 Think of pink salt as a mineral multivitamin—one that supports weight loss, wellness, and long-term health with every pinch.

Pink Salt vs. Table Salt

Salt is a staple in nearly every kitchen—but not all salt is created equal.

While both Himalayan pink salt and table salt contain sodium chloride as their base, their source, composition, processing, and health effects are drastically different. Understanding these differences is key to unlocking the benefits of the Pink Salt Trick Diet and making informed choices for your long-term wellness.

1. Source and Origin

- Himalayan Pink Salt is mined from ancient salt deposits deep within the Himalayan Mountains, primarily in the Khewra Salt Mine of Pakistan. These deposits formed millions of years ago from the evaporation of prehistoric seas and have remained untouched by modern pollution.
- Table Salt, by contrast, is typically harvested from modern seawater or underground salt domes. It undergoes heavy refining and chemical treatment before it reaches your table.

2. Processing and Additives

- Pink Salt is minimally processed. It's washed, crushed, and packaged without removing its natural minerals. It contains no additives, anti-caking agents, or bleaches.
- Table Salt is highly refined. In processing, nearly all natural minerals are stripped away. To prevent clumping, it's often treated with anti-caking agents, and in many countries, synthetic iodine is added to prevent iodine deficiency.

3. Mineral Content

- Pink Salt contains over 80 trace minerals including potassium, magnesium, calcium, iron, and zinc—each of which supports hydration, metabolism, and detoxification.
- Table Salt contains almost none of these beneficial trace minerals. It's made up of about 97–99% pure sodium chloride, making it more likely to disrupt your body's natural mineral balance when consumed in excess.

4. Taste and Culinary Experience

- Pink Salt offers a more rounded, earthy, and subtle flavor, thanks to its mineral complexity. Many chefs and wellness cooks prefer it for its enhanced taste and color.
- Table Salt has a sharper, more chemically "salty" flavor, and it's easy to overuse because it lacks complexity, often leading to excessive sodium intake.

♡ 5. Health Impact

Feature	Himalayan Pink Salt	Table Salt
Sodium Content	Slightly lower per gram	Higher per gram
Minerals	80+ trace minerals	Almost none
Processing	Unrefined, natural	Heavily refined, bleached
Additives	None	Anti-caking agents, added iodine
Health Impact	Supports hydration, metabolism, hormone balance	Can contribute to bloating, hypertension, and imbalance when overused
Supports Weight Loss?	☑ Yes, through mineral support and reduced water retention	✗ No, may promote water retention and cravings

💡 In Summary: Why Pink Salt Wins

Choosing Himalayan pink salt means:

- You're replacing lost minerals, not just adding sodium
- You're supporting natural detox and hydration
- You're enhancing your meals with clean, chemical-free seasoning
- You're practicing moderation with a more flavorful, satisfying salt

🧂 *The goal isn't to fear salt—it's to choose the right kind of salt. With pink salt, every pinch works with your body, not against it.*

How It Works for Weight Loss

At first glance, the idea that a small amount of salt in warm water could help with weight loss might sound far-fetched. But the Pink Salt Trick is not a gimmick—it's a simple, strategic tool based on how minerals interact with your body's metabolic systems.

Let's break down how this works.

1. Replenishes Essential Minerals for Fat Burning

Weight loss isn't just about "eating less." It's about how efficiently your body can:

- Digest food
- Convert nutrients into energy
- Regulate hormones and eliminate waste

These functions all depend on trace minerals like magnesium, potassium, sodium, calcium, and zinc—many of which are found in Himalayan pink salt.

When your body lacks these minerals, metabolism slows, digestion becomes sluggish, and fat is stored more easily.

Pink salt provides a daily, bioavailable source of these minerals, supporting:

- Hormonal balance
- Energy production
- Enzyme activation for fat breakdown

2. Balances Hydration and Reduces Bloating

Despite what many believe, proper salt intake doesn't cause water retention—imbalanced salt intake does.

When you drink pink salt water (especially in the morning), it helps:

- Restore electrolyte balance
- Flush out excess water held due to poor hydration
- Stimulate natural elimination through the bowels

As a result, many people experience:

- A flatter stomach
- Less puffiness in the face and hands
- Improved hydration at the cellular level

This is especially helpful during the detox phase of weight loss, when the body is shedding waste and recalibrating its systems.

3. Curbs Cravings and Stabilizes Blood Sugar

Mineral deficiencies are one of the most overlooked causes of cravings—especially for salty, sugary, or carb-heavy foods. When your body is missing key nutrients like magnesium or zinc, it sends urgent signals for food—often the wrong kind.

Daily pink salt intake helps reduce:

- Unnecessary snacking
- Blood sugar crashes
- Hormonal eating urges

You feel more satisfied between meals, making it easier to maintain a calorie deficit without feeling deprived.

🔥 4. Stimulates Digestive Enzymes and Gut Motility

When you drink pink salt water in the morning, you're giving your digestive system a wake-up call. The natural sodium content:

- Stimulates hydrochloric acid (HCl) in the stomach
- Aids bile production, breaking down fats
- Encourages peristalsis (the rhythmic movement of digestion)

The result? Better nutrient absorption, less gas and bloating, and improved gut efficiency.

A properly functioning digestive tract burns fat more effectively, and helps prevent fat storage from undigested food.

🧠 5. Supports Adrenal and Thyroid Health

Your adrenal glands (which regulate stress hormones) and thyroid (which controls metabolism) rely on trace minerals—especially sodium, iodine, magnesium, and selenium—to function properly.

Chronic stress, dieting, caffeine, and processed food deplete these minerals quickly.

By gently restoring them through daily pink salt use, you help:

- Stabilize cortisol (the belly fat hormone)
- Improve sleep and energy
- Normalize thyroid hormone output, which drives your metabolism

This mineral support is what makes the Pink Salt Trick especially powerful for women, whose hormones are often more sensitive to stress and nutrient imbalances.

📋 When and How to Use the Pink Salt Trick

The basic protocol:

1. Mix ¼–½ tsp of Himalayan pink salt in 8–12 oz of warm water
2. Drink first thing in the morning on an empty stomach
3. Wait at least 30 minutes before eating breakfast
4. Follow up with plenty of clean water throughout the day

Repeat daily throughout your 30-day meal plan, especially during the detox and fat-burning phases.

🧘 *Remember: This isn't a "quick fix." The trick works best when paired with clean eating, hydration, sleep, and consistency.*

⚠️ Safety Notes

- If you have hypertension, kidney issues, or are on a sodium-restricted plan, consult your doctor before starting.
- Always use food-grade, fine-grain Himalayan pink salt, not bath salts or coarse chunks.

🎯 In Summary

The Pink Salt Trick promotes weight loss by:

- Rebalancing minerals for efficient metabolism
- Reducing water retention and bloating
- Curbing cravings naturally
- Enhancing digestion and gut health

- Supporting stress management and hormone function

Detoxification Mechanism

A healthy body is naturally equipped to eliminate toxins—but in today's world, processed foods, stress, dehydration, and environmental exposure can overwhelm those systems. This is where Himalayan pink salt plays a key role in supporting and optimizing your body's detoxification process.

Let's explore how the Pink Salt Trick aids detox—gently, naturally, and effectively.

1. Encourages Daily Elimination

One of the primary ways your body eliminates waste is through the bowels. Many people unknowingly suffer from sluggish digestion, leading to:

- Bloating
- Fatigue
- Skin breakouts
- Weight retention

The Pink Salt Trick stimulates the gastrocolic reflex, a natural signal to your colon to begin moving waste when you consume warm fluids, especially in the morning.

When pink salt is added:

- It acts as an osmotic agent, drawing water into the intestines
- This softens stool and encourages gentle, regular bowel movements
- It helps flush out undigested waste and reduce harmful gut bacteria buildup

Many readers report feeling "lighter" and more energized within days of starting the salt flush.

2. Replenishes Detox-Supporting Minerals

Detoxification isn't just about removing waste—it's also about replenishing nutrients that support the liver, kidneys, and lymphatic system.

Himalayan pink salt provides critical minerals like:

- **Magnesium**, which supports liver enzyme activation
- **Calcium**, which binds to toxins in the gut
- **Potassium**, which regulates cellular hydration and electrolyte flow
- **Zinc & selenium**, which fuel antioxidant defense mechanisms

These minerals act like spark plugs for your detox organs, helping them break down and safely eliminate toxins more efficiently.

3. Promotes Lymphatic Drainage and Cellular Cleansing

Your lymphatic system is like the body's sanitation crew—it clears waste from tissues and transports it for removal. When your minerals are depleted or you're dehydrated, this system slows down.

Pink salt:

- Supports proper hydration, keeping lymph fluid moving
- Encourages cellular detox, allowing toxins to leave tissues more freely
- May reduce puffiness and water retention associated with stagnant lymph flow

When paired with light exercise or dry brushing, pink salt use can amplify lymphatic drainage, helping the body reset from the inside out.

⚡ 4. Boosts Liver and Kidney Efficiency

Your liver and kidneys work 24/7 to filter out toxins, hormones, and metabolic waste. But stress, medications, and poor diet can overburden these organs.

The trace minerals in Himalayan pink salt:

- Stimulate bile flow and liver enzyme activity
- Aid kidney filtration and reduce the workload on these organs
- Assist in neutralizing acidic waste that can accumulate from poor diet or dehydration

Many detox symptoms—like brain fog, fatigue, and irritability—are eased when these organs get the support they need from mineral-rich hydration.

♻ 5. Reduces "Toxic Weight"

What many people don't realize is that the body stores certain toxins in fat cells to protect vital organs. This is often called toxic weight—and it's why weight loss is difficult if your body feels too toxic to safely release stored fat.

By using pink salt to:

- Support daily elimination
- Reduce inflammation
- Replenish minerals
- Improve hydration

...you're signaling to your body: *"It's safe to let go."* And that's when fat burning accelerates naturally.

🛑 Detox Without Deprivation

Unlike harsh cleanses or juice fasts, the Pink Salt Trick doesn't force your body to detox. It gently supports what your body is already trying to do—flush toxins, balance fluids, and restore energy.

You don't need to starve. You don't need to suffer.

You just need a daily commitment to hydration, minerals, and clean eating—all of which are built into your 30-Day Pink Salt Meal Plan.

Appetite Control & Cravings Reduction

One of the biggest obstacles to sustainable weight loss isn't just what you eat—it's why you eat.

Cravings, emotional eating, constant snacking, and unstable hunger cues are all symptoms of an underlying imbalance in the body. The Pink Salt Trick helps correct these imbalances by restoring mineral levels, regulating hunger hormones, and reprogramming the body's natural appetite signals.

Let's explore how.

🧂 1. Mineral Deficiency = False Hunger

Cravings are often misunderstood as a lack of willpower—but in reality, they're usually a signal from the body that something important is missing.

When you're low on key minerals like:

- **Magnesium**
- **Zinc**
- **Potassium**
- **Sodium**

...your body may trigger strong urges for sugar, salt, or processed carbs to quickly compensate for the deficiency—even though those foods won't actually fix the problem.

Himalayan pink salt naturally supplies over 80 trace minerals that help:

- Satisfy true biological hunger
- Signal fullness more efficiently
- Stop the craving cycle before it starts

2. Stabilizes Hunger Hormones

Your hunger is regulated by hormones like ghrelin (the hunger hormone) and leptin (the fullness hormone). When these are out of sync—due to stress, poor sleep, or blood sugar fluctuations—you can feel constantly hungry, even after eating.

Here's how the Pink Salt Trick helps:

- Sodium and magnesium in pink salt support adrenal and thyroid function, which play a role in hormonal balance
- Drinking the pink salt flush in the morning prevents early blood sugar dips, which often lead to uncontrollable snacking later
- Restoring mineral balance helps your body release leptin more reliably, so you know when you're full

3. Reduces Sugar and Carb Cravings

Cravings for sweets and carbs are often a sign of unstable blood sugar or mineral imbalance.

The Pink Salt Trick:

- Provides minerals like magnesium and zinc that help regulate insulin
- Improves hydration, which is often misinterpreted by the brain as hunger
- Supports cortisol balance, reducing stress-eating triggers

Fun Fact: Many people who crave chocolate are actually low in magnesium—a key mineral found in pink salt.

4. Promotes Mindful Eating

By starting your day with a mineral-rich pink salt flush, you're also creating a pause before eating—giving your body time to:

- Wake up your digestive system
- Tune in to true hunger cues
- Avoid mindless morning snacking or overeating

This daily ritual naturally leads to greater awareness around food, helping you make better choices throughout the day.

5. Enhances Satiety from Meals

The minerals in pink salt improve nutrient absorption, which means:

- Your body gets more value from the food you eat
- You feel more satisfied with less
- You experience fewer between-meal crashes and hunger spikes

Combined with the balanced, high-fiber recipes in this book, the Pink Salt Trick helps turn every meal into a more complete, more fulfilling experience.

In Summary

The Pink Salt Trick helps control appetite and reduce cravings by:

- Replenishing essential minerals linked to hunger regulation
- Supporting hormonal balance
- Stabilizing blood sugar
- Encouraging mindful, intentional eating

When your body is nourished, hydrated, and mineralized, you'll be amazed how naturally your cravings fade—and how easy it becomes to say no to the foods that once felt irresistible.

Balancing Electrolytes & Boosting Metabolism

One of the most overlooked keys to natural, sustainable weight loss is electrolyte balance—and Himalayan pink salt plays a powerful role in keeping this delicate system in check.

Electrolytes are essential minerals that carry electrical charges and help regulate nearly every major function in your body, including:

- Metabolism
- Fat-burning enzymes
- Cellular hydration
- Muscle function
- Hormonal signaling

When your electrolytes are imbalanced, your metabolism slows, energy drops, and fat loss becomes harder than it needs to be.

💧 What Are Electrolytes—and Why Do They Matter?

The major electrolytes your body needs include:

- Sodium
- Potassium
- Magnesium
- Calcium
- Chloride

Together, they:

- Maintain fluid balance between cells
- Conduct nerve impulses that control digestion and metabolism
- Regulate thyroid and adrenal function, which drive fat-burning hormones
- Help convert food into usable energy (instead of storing it as fat)

When these minerals are too low—often due to restrictive dieting, intense exercise, caffeine, or stress—your body becomes dehydrated at the cellular level, leading to:

- Cravings
- Brain fog
- Sluggish metabolism
- Fat storage instead of fat burning

🧂 How Himalayan Pink Salt Restores Electrolyte Balance

Himalayan pink salt naturally provides:

- **Sodium**, to help maintain blood volume and cell hydration
- **Magnesium**, which activates over 300 metabolic enzymes
- **Potassium**, to balance sodium levels and support heart rhythm
- **Calcium**, which assists in fat-burning and muscle contractions

This mineral-rich profile helps your body retain the right amount of water—not too much, not too little. As a result, you'll:

- Feel more energized
- Eliminate bloating and puffiness
- Improve metabolic efficiency

💡 *Unlike processed table salt, pink salt supports hydration and energy without causing water retention or mineral imbalance.*

🔥 The Metabolism Connection

Your metabolism isn't just one thing—it's a collection of processes that turn food into fuel, burn stored fat, and keep your body functioning smoothly.

Here's how pink salt helps boost it:

- Activates digestive enzymes that speed up nutrient breakdown
- Supports thyroid health, which controls your basal metabolic rate (BMR)
- Improves adrenal support, preventing stress-related slowdowns in fat burning
- Enhances mitochondrial function, which is where calories are converted into usable energy

When electrolyte levels are optimized, your body becomes a fat-burning machine—rather than storing energy as fat due to stress, dehydration, or confusion in hunger signals.

🔎 Signs of Electrolyte Imbalance That Pink Salt Can Help Improve

- Constant fatigue despite rest
- Cramping, muscle weakness, or brain fog
- Chronic bloating or water retention
- Dizziness when standing up quickly
- Poor workout recovery
- Intense cravings for salty or sugary snacks

If any of these sound familiar, there's a strong chance your body is low on essential minerals—and the Pink Salt Trick is your first, simplest step toward correcting it.

🔑 Consistency Is Key

The Pink Salt Trick isn't a one-time detox—it's a daily support system that:

- Replenishes electrolytes lost through sweat, stress, and diet
- Keeps your metabolism functioning at its peak
- Prepares your body to handle natural weight loss without burnout

And when paired with the right meals (which this book provides), it becomes even more effective.

Scientific Insights and Evidence

While Himalayan pink salt may seem like a trendy wellness product, its health-supportive properties are rooted in biochemistry, mineral science, and human physiology. This section explores the scientific principles behind the Pink Salt Trick and explains why it works—not just anecdotally, but mechanistically.

Let's take a closer look at the research-backed foundations of this natural approach to weight loss, detox, and metabolic support.

🍬 1. Trace Minerals and Metabolic Function

Minerals such as magnesium, zinc, calcium, potassium, and sodium are essential for:

- Enzyme activity
- Thyroid hormone production
- Mitochondrial energy generation
- Glucose metabolism
- Appetite regulation

A 2019 review in Nutrients journal emphasized that mineral deficiencies are directly linked to impaired fat metabolism, insulin resistance, and increased inflammation—all factors that hinder weight loss.

By restoring these trace minerals daily via pink salt, the body is better equipped to:

- Burn calories efficiently
- Process carbohydrates without insulin spikes
- Balance hormones involved in appetite and energy regulation

💧 2. Sodium Intake and Hydration—A Balanced View

Sodium is often vilified in health conversations, but context matters.

According to research published in the *Journal of Clinical Hypertension*, low sodium diets can impair hydration, reduce blood volume, and disrupt adrenal function, especially in active individuals or those under stress.

The controlled use of natural, mineral-rich salt—like the Pink Salt Trick—helps:

- Support fluid balance at the cellular level
- Optimize nutrient transport into cells
- Prevent dehydration-related fatigue and brain fog

☑️ *Conclusion:* When consumed in moderation and alongside proper hydration, pink salt supports, rather than sabotages, long-term health.

🍬 3. Gut Health and Salt-Induced Enzyme Activation

Your digestive efficiency has a huge impact on weight loss. Without proper stomach acid and bile flow, nutrients aren't absorbed and food ferments, causing bloating, toxicity, and fat storage.

Studies have shown that sodium chloride stimulates hydrochloric acid (HCl) production in the stomach. Pink salt, in particular, due to its trace mineral profile, may also support the release of digestive enzymes, according to findings in *Frontiers in Physiology* (2020).

Improved digestion = better fat breakdown = more efficient metabolism.

🧠 4. Pink Salt and Stress Reduction

Chronic stress drives up cortisol—a hormone that causes:

- Belly fat retention
- Blood sugar imbalances
- Cravings for sugary or salty foods

Electrolytes like magnesium and sodium are crucial for adrenal function. A well-mineralized body is more resilient under stress, keeping cortisol in check and preventing emotional eating.

A study published in *Biological Trace Element Research* (2018) linked trace mineral supplementation to lower cortisol levels, improved sleep, and greater emotional regulation—all key to successful weight loss.

🧪 5. Detoxification Support

Detoxification is a biological process—handled by your liver, kidneys, lymph, and skin. But without the right cofactors (like minerals), these systems slow down.

Scientific evidence shows that minerals such as selenium, magnesium, and zinc play a vital role in:

- Liver enzyme function
- Glutathione production (the body's master antioxidant)
- Heavy metal removal and bile processing

Himalayan pink salt contributes to these processes naturally—no pills or extreme cleanses required.

🧂 6. Beyond Anecdote—Real Observations

Though large-scale clinical trials specifically on Himalayan pink salt are limited, anecdotal evidence combined with existing studies on mineral rebalancing, sodium regulation, and detoxification offer a strong scientific basis for its use.

Thousands of individuals report:

- Reduced bloating and puffiness
- Stabilized hunger and fewer cravings
- Easier, more regular elimination
- Better hydration and energy
- Steady fat loss when combined with clean eating

Misconceptions & Cautions

As interest in Himalayan pink salt and natural detox methods grows, so do myths, misunderstandings, and exaggerated claims. While the Pink Salt Trick is safe, gentle, and effective when used correctly, it's important to separate fact from fiction—and understand where caution is necessary.

This section addresses the most common misconceptions and outlines clear safety guidelines, so you can move forward informed and empowered.

❌ Misconception #1: "All salt is bad for you."

This is one of the most pervasive myths in health and weight loss culture. While excessive intake of refined table salt can increase the risk of hypertension and fluid retention, not all salt is created equal.

Himalayan pink salt:

- Is unprocessed and mineral-rich
- Supports hydration and electrolyte balance
- Contains less sodium per teaspoon than table salt due to its crystal structure

When used in moderation, it becomes a healing ally, not a health hazard.

⚠️ *Caution:* People with pre-existing heart, kidney, or blood pressure conditions should always consult a physician before increasing any salt intake.

❌ Misconception #2: "The Pink Salt Trick is a miracle weight loss cure."

Let's be clear: No single ingredient or method—not even pink salt—can replace a balanced diet, movement, hydration, and rest. The Pink Salt Trick is a supportive tool, not a magic pill.

It works by:

- Enhancing digestion
- Rebalancing hydration
- Reducing cravings
- Supporting natural detox

When paired with the 30-day plan provided in this book, these small changes compound into significant results.

✘ Misconception #3: "More salt = faster results."

More is not better. Using too much pink salt—even if it's natural—can lead to:

- Dehydration
- Electrolyte imbalance
- Bloating or diarrhea
- Elevated blood pressure in sensitive individuals

☑ The solution? Stick to safe amounts:

- ¼ to ½ teaspoon of fine-grain, food-grade pink salt in 8–12 oz of warm water once per day is all you need.

✘ Misconception #4: "Pink salt detoxes your body on its own."

The truth is: your body detoxes itself every day—through your liver, kidneys, gut, lymph, and skin.

Pink salt doesn't "flush" toxins like a laxative or cleanse would. Instead, it:

- Supports the organs that naturally detoxify
- Enhances digestion and regularity
- Replenishes minerals required for cellular repair and waste removal

✘ Misconception #5: "If I feel tired or bloated, the salt isn't working."

In the first few days of the Pink Salt Trick, some people may experience:

- Mild fatigue
- Loose stools
- Slight headache

This is often a temporary detox response, especially if your body is adjusting to better hydration or eliminating old waste.

💡 *Tip: Ease into the process with plenty of water and fiber-rich meals from this cookbook.*

🧘 Guidelines for Safe & Effective Use

- Always use fine-grain, food-grade Himalayan pink salt—not bath salts or decorative blocks
- Start with ¼ teaspoon daily, increase to ½ teaspoon only if tolerated well
- Drink the mixture on an empty stomach, preferably in the morning
- Wait 30 minutes before eating to allow digestion to activate
- Follow with clean, mineral-rich meals for optimal results
- Stay well-hydrated throughout the day to support kidney and bowel function

🚫 Who Should Not Use the Pink Salt Trick Without Medical Advice

- Individuals with high blood pressure or heart conditions

- Anyone with kidney disease or electrolyte imbalance
- Pregnant or breastfeeding women
- People on sodium-restricted diets or taking diuretics
- Children under 12 years old

✅ In Summary

The Pink Salt Trick is simple, natural, and effective—but like any wellness tool, it should be used wisely and responsibly.

When practiced with awareness and paired with nourishing food, hydration, and movement, this technique can:

- Support healthy weight loss
- Rebalance your body
- Help you feel clearer, lighter, and more energized

📘 *It's not a shortcut—it's a smart step toward a balanced, sustainable lifestyle.*

How Much Pink Salt is Safe to Consume?

When it comes to the Pink Salt Trick, balance is everything. Himalayan pink salt is a natural source of vital minerals, but like anything—even water or sunshine—too much of a good thing can become problematic if not used mindfully.

This section will help you understand safe daily limits, how to adjust your intake based on individual needs, and when to seek medical advice.

✅ General Safety Guidelines

The recommended safe daily intake of sodium for most healthy adults is:

- 1,500–2,300 mg of sodium per day, as per the American Heart Association and WHO.

Himalayan pink salt is approximately 98% sodium chloride, which means:

- 1/4 teaspoon = ~500–550 mg of sodium
- 1/2 teaspoon = ~1,100–1,200 mg of sodium

➡ For the Pink Salt Trick:

- Start with 1/4 teaspoon in 8–12 oz of warm water, once daily, preferably in the morning on an empty stomach.
- If well tolerated after several days, increase to 1/2 teaspoon max per day, if needed.

💡 *This allows you to benefit from mineral replenishment without exceeding safe sodium limits—especially when paired with a low-processed, whole-food diet as outlined in this cookbook.*

⚖ Adjusting Based on Individual Needs

Everyone's body is different. Consider the following when determining your ideal pink salt intake:

🏃 Higher Needs (closer to 1/2 tsp daily):

- Active individuals or athletes who sweat frequently
- People transitioning off processed foods (which often spike cravings during mineral withdrawal)
- Those practicing intermittent fasting (for electrolyte support)

- Individuals living in hot, humid climates

🧂 Lower Needs (stay at 1/4 tsp or less):

- Sedentary lifestyles
- Diets already high in sodium (from cheese, deli meats, canned goods)
- Individuals with a family history of heart or kidney issues
- Anyone on medications that affect electrolyte levels (e.g., diuretics)

🩺 When to Consult a Doctor First

You must speak with a healthcare provider before beginning the Pink Salt Trick if you:

- Have high blood pressure, heart disease, or kidney problems
- Are on a sodium-restricted diet
- Are pregnant, breastfeeding, or taking prescription medications that affect hydration or minerals
- Experience symptoms like dizziness, swelling, or palpitations during use

⚠ *While the Pink Salt Trick is gentle, it does introduce a mineral shift in your body—so if you have a medical condition, always get professional clearance.*

💧 Hydration Is Non-Negotiable

Salt draws water. To ensure safe and effective results:

- Drink plenty of clean water throughout the day (at least 8–10 cups for most adults)
- Do not consume pink salt without water or during dehydration
- Watch for signs of electrolyte imbalance such as extreme thirst, dry mouth, dizziness, or unusual fatigue

💧 *Think of pink salt as a mineral conductor—without water, its benefits can't be delivered where they're needed.*

🧂 Other Ways to Use Pink Salt Throughout the Day

While the morning flush is the primary technique, you can also incorporate pink salt into:

- Meals (season lightly—use it to enhance, not oversaturate)
- Hydration drinks after workouts
- Homemade broth or soup recipes in this book
- Mineral-rich baths (topical use, not for consumption)

Just remember: total intake should remain under 2,300 mg sodium per day for most healthy adults—including all food and drink sources combined.

🧂 In Summary

How much pink salt is safe?

→ ¼ to ½ teaspoon per day, when dissolved in water, used mindfully, and paired with adequate hydration and a clean diet.

This amount:

- Supports metabolism
- Replenishes electrolytes
- Aids detoxification
- Curbs cravings—without compromising safety

The key is consistency, not excess. Trust the process, listen to your body, and follow the plan laid out in this book for optimal results.

The Pink Salt Morning Flush Explained

Now that you understand the power of Himalayan pink salt and how it supports weight loss, detox, and metabolic health, it's time to put it into practice.

Enter your new wellness ritual: **The Pink Salt Morning Flush.**

This simple daily habit is at the heart of the Pink Salt Trick Diet. It's designed to wake up your digestive system, rehydrate your body, replenish minerals, and trigger fat-burning processes—all before your first bite of breakfast.

Let's break it down.

🧂 What Is the Pink Salt Morning Flush?

It's a warm, mineral-rich drink made from Himalayan pink salt and clean water, consumed on an empty stomach first thing in the morning.

The goal?

To jumpstart your day by:

- Flushing out toxins
- Rehydrating your cells
- Stimulating digestion
- Reducing bloating
- Enhancing energy and focus
- Rebalancing electrolytes after a night of fasting

🧂 How to Prepare It

Ingredients:

- ¼ to ½ teaspoon of fine-grain food-grade Himalayan pink salt
- 8 to 12 ounces (1 to 1½ cups) of warm, filtered water
- (Not hot and not cold—think gently warmed to body temperature)

Instructions:

1. Dissolve the pink salt completely in the warm water.

2. Stir gently until the water is clear and salt is fully mixed in.

3. Drink it slowly and mindfully—don't chug.

4. Wait 20–30 minutes before eating or drinking anything else.

Optional: Add a squeeze of fresh lemon juice for added detox and flavor benefits.

⏰ When to Take It

- Best consumed immediately upon waking
- Before coffee, tea, or breakfast
- After brushing your teeth (to avoid tasting salt first thing)

Make it a daily morning ritual—consistent timing is key to results.

💡 What Happens in Your Body After the Flush?

Within 20–30 minutes, you may notice:

- A gentle urge to go to the bathroom (a good sign—it means your digestion is waking up)

- A decrease in morning bloating or puffiness
- A clearer mind and lighter feeling
- Fewer cravings later in the day
- More consistent energy without caffeine crashes

This is your body hydrating, balancing, and cleansing before food even enters the system.

🚫 What Not to Do

- Don't drink it with food or after meals—it's most effective on an empty stomach
- Don't use coarse salt chunks (they may not dissolve fully or measure accurately)
- Don't overdo the salt—stick to ¼–½ teaspoon max per day
- Don't skip hydration—drink clean water throughout the day to support mineral movement

📅 How Often Should You Do the Flush?

→ Daily during the 30-Day Pink Salt Trick Plan in this book

→ Continue 3–5 days a week afterward for maintenance and long-term wellness

This isn't just a detox—it's a foundational habit that helps set the tone for the rest of your day, both physically and mentally.

⚠️ Possible Early Reactions

Especially during the first few days, you may experience:

- Mild loose stools or more frequent bathroom trips
- Slight headaches (usually from detox or dehydration—drink more water)
- Temporary fatigue as the body resets and clears out stored waste

✅ These are normal transitional symptoms and typically resolve within 2–4 days. Listen to your body, rest if needed, and stay hydrated.

🧘 Make It a Mindful Ritual

Treat the Pink Salt Morning Flush as more than a drink—let it become a moment of calm, care, and commitment to your well-being.

Light a candle, take deep breaths, write a goal for the day—whatever helps you start from a place of empowerment.

CHAPTER 2: GETTING STARTED WITH THE PINK SALT LIFESTYLE

Preparing Your Pantry

Before beginning your 30-day journey with the Pink Salt Trick Diet, it's important to set yourself up for success—starting with your pantry. A well-stocked, intentionally organized kitchen removes guesswork, reduces temptation, and makes it easier to build meals that align with your weight loss and wellness goals.

This isn't about throwing everything out. It's about clearing space for the foods and tools that support your transformation.

Let's walk through the process, step-by-step.

🖌 Step 1: Declutter and Detox Your Pantry

Just like your body, your pantry may be holding onto things it no longer needs. Begin by checking for:

- Expired products
- Highly processed foods (chips, sugary cereals, boxed dinners)
- Refined white sugars and flours
- Low-quality table salt (which will be replaced by pink salt)
- Artificial additives (MSG, food dyes, hydrogenated oils)

You don't need to go cold turkey—but begin by removing or reducing items that won't serve your goals during this 30-day reset.

Tip: Donate unopened non-perishables to a local shelter if they no longer fit your nutrition plan.

🧂 Step 2: Stock the Essentials for the Pink Salt Lifestyle

Here's what to keep on hand for preparing delicious, clean, pink salt–enhanced meals:

🧂 Salts & Seasonings

- Fine-grain Himalayan pink salt (daily flush & cooking)
- Black pepper (fresh ground)
- Turmeric
- Smoked paprika
- Garlic powder
- Onion powder
- Italian herb blend
- Cumin, ginger, cinnamon
- Chili flakes or cayenne (optional for thermogenic boost)

🥦 Whole Food Staples

- Brown rice, wild rice, or quinoa
- Rolled oats or steel-cut oats
- Lentils (red, green, or brown)
- Chickpeas, black beans, white beans
- Whole grain or legume-based pasta
- Unsweetened nut butter (almond, peanut, sunflower)

🥑 Healthy Fats

- Extra virgin olive oil
- Avocado oil (for high-heat cooking)
- Coconut oil (optional for flavor variation)

- Raw nuts & seeds (chia, flax, walnuts, almonds, pumpkin seeds)

🥫 Canned & Jarred Goods (Low Sodium Preferred)

- Coconut milk
- Crushed tomatoes
- Tuna or salmon (packed in water or olive oil)
- Nut milk (almond, oat, or coconut—unsweetened)
- Vegetable or bone broth (no added MSG or preservatives)

🌿 Superfoods & Add-Ins

- Apple cider vinegar (for metabolism support)
- Ground flaxseed or chia seeds
- Nutritional yeast (for vegan-friendly protein + flavor)
- Herbal teas (peppermint, ginger, chamomile, dandelion root)
- Organic lemon juice (or fresh lemons)

❄️ Step 3: Freezer-Friendly Staples

Stock your freezer with clean, go-to proteins and backup veggies:

- Frozen berries (for smoothies or breakfasts)
- Frozen spinach, broccoli, or cauliflower
- Frozen grilled chicken, shrimp, or tofu
- Pre-cooked brown rice or quinoa packs
- Veggie-based burger patties (read labels for clean ingredients)

🥗 Step 4: Fresh Weekly Picks

Plan to rotate in weekly fresh ingredients:

- Leafy greens (kale, spinach, romaine, arugula)
- Cruciferous veggies (broccoli, cabbage, cauliflower)
- Sweet potatoes, zucchini, bell peppers, onions
- Avocados, lemons, apples, bananas, cucumbers
- Fresh herbs (parsley, cilantro, basil)

🧰 Step 5: Tools That Help You Succeed

You don't need a fancy kitchen, but these basic tools make prepping Pink Salt meals much easier:

- Large water bottle or glass jug (for staying hydrated)
- Mason jars or glass containers (for soaking oats or meal prep)
- High-speed blender (for smoothies and soups)
- Nonstick pan and baking sheet (for roasting veggies or protein)
- Steamer basket (for gentle cooking)
- Measuring spoons and digital scale (optional, for precision)

🧂 <u>Final Pantry Tip: Keep It Visible and Inspiring</u>

Organize your healthy ingredients so they're easy to see and reach.

Put your Himalayan pink salt in a small glass container with a scoop near your kettle or water station as a visual reminder to start your day right.

📌 *The more effortless your environment, the more consistent your results.*

Recommended Kitchen Tools

Eating well doesn't require a commercial kitchen—just the right tools to make prepping, cooking, and portioning both enjoyable and efficient.

This list includes simple, accessible tools to help you prepare the 60+ pink salt recipes and stick to your 30-day plan with ease.

Think of this as your essentials checklist for flavorful meals, consistent habits, and less time stressing in the kitchen.

🔍 Cooking Tools

☑ **Nonstick Skillet or Ceramic Frying Pan**

For sautéing vegetables, eggs, tofu, or lean proteins with minimal oil.

☑ **Medium & Large Saucepan**

Ideal for boiling grains, simmering soups, or cooking legumes.

☑ **Baking Sheet or Sheet Pan**

For roasting vegetables, chickpeas, or protein-packed one-pan dinners.

☑ **Steamer Basket or Insert**

Preserves nutrients while steaming greens, fish, or sweet potatoes.

☑ **Rice Cooker or Instant Pot (Optional)**

Saves time for cooking rice, quinoa, and lentils perfectly with zero babysitting.

🔪 Prep Tools

☑ **Sharp Chef's Knife**

A quality knife saves time and helps you prep efficiently and safely.

☑ **Cutting Boards (2)**

One for produce, one for proteins—essential for food safety.

☑ **Measuring Cups and Spoons**

For precise portion control, especially with pink salt and dressings.

☑ **Microplane or Grater**

Great for zesting lemons, grating ginger, or adding garlic without fuss.

☑ **Salad Spinner**

Makes leafy greens quick to wash and dry—so you actually use them.

🥣 Mixing & Storage

☑ **Mixing Bowls (Multiple Sizes)**

For meal prep, tossing salads, or mixing protein batters.

☑ **Glass Meal Prep Containers (with Lids)**

Portion out lunches or store leftovers. Glass is safer than plastic for reheating.

☑ **Mason Jars or Smoothie Bottles**

Perfect for overnight oats, chia pudding, infused waters, or homemade dressings.

🥣 Blending & Hydration

☑ High-Speed Blender

Essential for smoothies, soups, pink salt electrolyte drinks, and healthy sauces.

☑ Handheld Immersion Blender (Optional)

Blends soups and dressings right in the pot—no pouring or extra cleanup.

☑ Large Reusable Water Bottle or Pitcher

Keeps you on track with your hydration goals throughout the day.

🧂 Pink Salt Essentials

☑ Small Glass Jar or Salt Cellar

Store your Himalayan pink salt within easy reach near your kettle or stove.

☑ Electric or Gooseneck Kettle

For preparing your Pink Salt Morning Flush quickly and consistently.

📝 Optional but Helpful Tools

- Digital Kitchen Scale (for precision and portion awareness)
- Spiralizer (for zucchini noodles and veggie-forward meals)
- Air Fryer (for crisping veggies or proteins with minimal oil)
- Food Processor (for energy bites, hummus, or cauliflower rice)

🧘 Final Tip: Start With What You Have

Don't feel pressure to buy everything at once. Many recipes in this book can be made with just a knife, pan, blender, and bowl. Build your toolkit gradually based on your needs and preferences.

📌 *The goal isn't perfection—it's progress, simplicity, and sustainability.*

Shopping List for the First Week

Set yourself up for success with clean, nutrient-dense foods that align with the Pink Salt Trick lifestyle.

This curated list is designed to support your first 7 days of the 30-day plan, including breakfast, lunch, dinner, snacks, and your daily Pink Salt Flush. It's organized by category for easy grocery runs and pantry prep.

🧂 Minerals & Essentials

- Himalayan pink salt (fine-grain, food-grade)
- Fresh lemons (4–6)
- Filtered water (or access to clean drinking water)

🥬 Fresh Vegetables & Greens

- Spinach (fresh or baby, 2–3 handfuls)
- Kale or Swiss chard (1 bunch)
- Romaine or arugula (1 head or bag)
- Broccoli (2 crowns or 1 bag florets)
- Cauliflower (1 medium head)
- Zucchini (2)
- Bell peppers (2–3 mixed colors)
- Red onion (2)
- Garlic (1 bulb)

- Cherry or grape tomatoes (1 pint)
- Carrots (3–5)
- Avocados (2–3)
- Sweet potatoes (2–4 medium)
- Cucumber (1–2)
- Fresh herbs: cilantro, parsley, basil (1 bunch each)

🍉 Fresh Fruits

- Apples (4–5)
- Bananas (3–5)
- Berries (blueberries, strawberries, or raspberries – 1–2 cups total)
- Grapefruit or oranges (2–3)
- Frozen mango or pineapple (for smoothies – 1 bag)
- Lemons (extra for flushing + recipes)

🥫 Pantry Staples

- Rolled oats or steel-cut oats
- Brown rice, wild rice, or quinoa
- Lentils (red or green – 1 bag or 2 cans)
- Chickpeas (1–2 cans or dried)
- Black beans (1 can)
- Chia seeds
- Ground flaxseeds
- Extra virgin olive oil
- Avocado oil (optional, for cooking)
- Apple cider vinegar (raw, unfiltered)
- Nut butter (unsweetened almond or peanut)
- Coconut milk (1 can, full-fat or lite)
- Vegetable broth or low-sodium chicken broth (1 carton)
- Crushed tomatoes (1 can)
- Unsweetened nut milk (almond, oat, or coconut)
- Low-sodium tuna or salmon (1 can or pouch)

🥜 Nuts, Seeds & Snacks

- Raw almonds or walnuts (¼–½ cup)
- Pumpkin seeds or sunflower seeds
- Hummus (store-bought or ingredients to make your own)
- Rice cakes or whole grain crackers (optional, minimal ingredients)

🧄 Spices & Condiments

- Black pepper
- Smoked paprika
- Ground turmeric
- Ground cumin
- Cinnamon
- Dried Italian herbs or oregano
- Chili flakes (optional)
- Nutritional yeast (optional, for flavor and nutrients)
- Dijon mustard (optional for dressings)

❄️ Freezer Staples

- Frozen spinach or kale (1 bag, for smoothies or soups)
- Frozen mixed berries (1 bag)
- Frozen broccoli or green beans
- Frozen grilled chicken strips or tofu cubes

🥚 Protein Options

(Choose based on dietary preference)

- Eggs (1 dozen)

- Chicken breast or thighs (1–2 lbs)
- Salmon fillet or canned wild salmon
- Tofu or tempeh (1–2 blocks)
- Greek yogurt (plain, unsweetened – optional)

🧘 Optional Boosters

- Herbal teas: peppermint, chamomile, dandelion, or ginger
- Raw honey (for optional use in tea or dressings)
- Coconut aminos or low-sodium tamari (for stir-fries)

📝 Pro Tips for Success

- Plan 2–3 batch-cook sessions during the week to prep grains, roasted veggies, or proteins ahead.
- Stick to whole, unprocessed options as much as possible—read labels for added sugars and sodium.
- Prioritize hydration: Keep lemons and pink salt accessible near your water station.

Reading Food Labels & Sodium Awareness

Even with the healthiest intentions, hidden sodium and artificial additives can sneak into your meals and undermine your progress. That's why reading food labels isn't just a good habit—it's a key part of the Pink Salt Trick Diet.

This section will teach you how to decode food packaging, avoid sodium overload, and make smart choices that support natural detox, hydration, and sustainable weight loss.

🧂 Why Sodium Awareness Matters

While Himalayan pink salt, used in moderation, supports your health, most processed foods are loaded with refined salt (table salt)—which contains:

- No trace minerals
- Anti-caking chemicals
- Excess sodium that may lead to bloating, water retention, or elevated blood pressure

During the 30-Day Pink Salt Trick Diet, your goal is to:

- Control your sodium source (you choose pink salt)
- Keep total daily sodium under 2,300 mg
- Avoid sodium that comes from packaged, refined, or fast foods

📑 How to Read Food Labels for Sodium Clues

Here's a step-by-step guide to understanding the Nutrition Facts Panel on packaged foods:

1. Look at the Serving Size

Check how many servings are in the package—and how many you're actually consuming. Sodium is listed per serving, not per container.

2. Check Sodium Content (mg)

Look for the line that says "Sodium."

- Aim for 140 mg or less per serving (low sodium)
- Avoid anything with 400 mg or more per serving

🍲 *Example: If a soup has 780 mg of sodium per serving and you eat 2 servings, that's 1,560 mg in one meal—almost your full day's limit.*

3. Scan the Ingredient List

Ingredients are listed by weight, from most to least.

🚫 Watch out for these high-sodium ingredients:

- Monosodium glutamate (MSG)
- Sodium nitrate/nitrite
- Sodium benzoate
- Disodium phosphate
- Baking soda or baking powder (can be fine in moderation)
- Anything "flavored," "instant," or "seasoned"
- Broths or bouillons with "hydrolyzed" or "autolyzed" anything

✅ Look for clean, minimal-ingredient labels with herbs, spices, and real food words you recognize.

🛒 Tips for Smarter Shopping

- Choose "low sodium" or "no added salt" versions of canned beans, vegetables, or broths
- Rinse canned foods (like beans or tuna) under water for 10–15 seconds to remove up to 40% of sodium
- Cook from scratch when possible—it gives you full control over what goes in your body
- Use pink salt only during meal prep or in your flush—not on top of already-salty packaged foods
- Avoid "flavor enhancers" or seasoning blends that don't list their exact sodium content

⚠️ Watch Your Sodium Triggers

Even "healthy" foods can carry hidden salt. Be extra cautious with:

- Deli meats and plant-based sausages
- Salad dressings and condiments
- Sauces (especially soy sauce, teriyaki, BBQ, etc.)
- Nut butters and protein bars
- Pre-made frozen "healthy" meals

✅ In Summary: What to Look For

When reading labels:

- 140 mg sodium or less per serving is ideal
- Short ingredient lists with real, whole food names
- Low or no preservatives (especially sodium-based ones)
- Choose unsalted or lightly salted versions and season them yourself with pink salt

🧂 *The less salt you allow others to add to your food, the more power you have to control your health and results.*

Portion Sizes & Serving Tips

One of the keys to lasting weight loss is not just what you eat—but how much. Even healthy, mineral-rich foods can stall your progress if portion sizes are too large or unbalanced.

This section helps you tune into your body's hunger cues, make smart serving decisions, and learn how to eat intuitively but intentionally within the Pink Salt Trick Diet.

❂ Why Portion Control Matters

When you're eating nourishing whole foods seasoned with Himalayan pink salt, it's easy to think, "I can eat as much as I want." But for optimal results, we must:

- Respect our body's true hunger and fullness signals
- Avoid overeating—even clean, homemade meals
- Prevent hidden calorie creep from sauces, oils, or snacks
- Train your metabolism to use food as fuel, not excess storage

🍽 *Portion control is about awareness—not restriction.*

❂ Start With the 80% Rule

Eat until you're about 80% full, not stuffed. Your brain takes about 15–20 minutes to register fullness. Pause during meals to breathe, chew thoroughly, and check in with how you feel.

🍽 Smart Serving Tips by Meal

🥣 Breakfast

- Use a small bowl or jar for oatmeal, smoothies, or parfaits
- Add protein + healthy fat to control blood sugar and fullness
- Stick to 1 serving of fruit—avoid doubling portions unintentionally

🍲 Lunch & Dinner

a. Divide your plate:

- ½ vegetables
- ¼ lean protein
- ¼ complex carbs

b. Use a salad plate instead of a dinner plate to avoid overserving

c. Limit oils and dressings to 1–2 tablespoons total per meal

🥣 Snacks

- Pre-portion nuts, trail mix, or hummus instead of snacking from the container
- Choose nutrient-dense, low-calorie snacks (chia pudding, roasted chickpeas, sliced cucumbers with pink salt)
- Avoid snacking when bored—pause and drink water first

⚖ Mindful Eating Practices

- Sit down to eat—no screens, no multitasking
- Chew slowly and savor each bite
- Rest your utensils between bites
- Start meals with water or a veggie-based soup to help prevent overeating
- Use small plates and bowls for natural portion reduction

🍽 Batch Cooking? Pre-Portion to Stay on Track

When meal prepping:

- Use glass meal containers to portion out individual servings
- Store grains, proteins, and sauces separately to control balance and freshness
- Label containers with meal names or days to reduce decision fatigue

Hydration and the Role of Water

If Himalayan pink salt is the spark, then water is the fuel. Together, they create the internal environment your body needs to burn fat, flush toxins, boost energy, and support digestion. That's why hydration is a pillar of the Pink Salt Trick Diet—and not something to overlook.

This section explains why water plays such a crucial role, how it works in harmony with pink salt, and how to stay properly hydrated throughout your 30-day journey (and beyond).

💧 Why Hydration Is Essential

Your body is made up of 60–70% water, and nearly every system depends on it. Without proper hydration, no diet—no matter how clean—will work optimally.

Here's what water does for you:

- Regulates body temperature
- Supports digestion and nutrient absorption
- Helps flush out waste and toxins through the liver and kidneys
- Promotes healthy skin, joints, and muscle recovery
- Aids in appetite control and energy regulation

🧂 How Pink Salt and Water Work Together

Himalayan pink salt is rich in electrolytes—like sodium, magnesium, and potassium—which help your body retain the right amount of water in the right places.

Here's how the Pink Salt Trick enhances hydration:

- Helps water enter cells more efficiently (cellular hydration)
- Prevents overhydration and electrolyte dilution, which can cause fatigue
- Balances fluid retention—keeping just what your body needs
- Reduces symptoms like brain fog, dizziness, or water bloating

💡 *When your minerals are balanced, you hydrate more efficiently—less swelling, more energy, and improved digestion.*

🥤 How Much Water Should You Drink Daily?

There's no one-size-fits-all, but here's a simple formula:

Your weight (in pounds) ÷ 2 = ounces of water per day

→ Example: If you weigh 160 lbs, aim for about 80 oz (10 cups) of water daily.

Increase your intake if you:

- Exercise regularly
- Live in a hot/humid climate
- Drink coffee or alcohol
- Are detoxing or flushing with pink salt

✅ *Consistency matters more than volume. Spread your intake throughout the day instead of chugging large amounts at once.*

⏰ When to Drink Water

- Upon waking → with your Pink Salt Flush
- Before meals → 15–30 minutes prior to reduce overeating

- Between meals → to sustain energy and metabolism
- After workouts → to replenish electrolytes and reduce soreness
- Before bed → just a few sips (don't overdo it late at night)

✗ Signs of Dehydration to Watch For

Even mild dehydration can stall weight loss and increase cravings. Stay alert for:

- Dry mouth or cracked lips
- Headaches or fatigue
- Dizziness or light-headedness
- Constipation
- Dark yellow urine
- Sugar or salt cravings

✓ Hydration Tips for Success

- Carry a refillable water bottle throughout the day
- Infuse water with lemon, cucumber, mint, or berries for flavor
- Set phone reminders or use hydration apps if you tend to forget
- Keep water visible—on your desk, counter, or nightstand
- Drink water before reaching for snacks—many cravings are actually thirst signals

Supplements & Synergistic Superfoods

While the Pink Salt Trick lays a strong mineral foundation, your body may benefit even more from a few carefully chosen additions. These come in two forms: supplements, when needed, and superfoods that naturally enhance the diet's detox, fat-burning, and energy-boosting effects.

Let's explore how to use each—safely and intentionally.

💊 Do You Need Supplements?

Most people following the Pink Salt Trick Diet won't require supplements. The Himalayan pink salt you're using already provides sodium, magnesium, calcium, iron, and more than 80 trace minerals.

However, you might consider a supplement if you:

- Have diagnosed deficiencies (like iron, magnesium, or vitamin D)
- Experience adrenal fatigue or hormonal imbalances
- Follow a vegan, keto, or highly restrictive diet
- Suffer from sluggish digestion or chronic fatigue

If so, you may benefit from magnesium glycinate or citrate for sleep and muscle relaxation, a high-quality vitamin D3 with K2 for immunity and metabolism, or a daily probiotic for digestion. Some people also use omega-3 supplements from fish or algae oil to fight inflammation and improve heart health. And for those dealing with stress or cravings, adaptogenic herbs like ashwagandha or rhodiola may support adrenal function.

Note: Always consult your doctor or a nutritionist before starting any supplement, especially if you're on medication or managing a health condition.

🪶 Synergistic Superfoods to Boost Your Results

Whole foods often outperform pills, especially when eaten consistently. Here are some simple, powerful ingredients to weave into your meals:

- **Leafy greens** like spinach, kale, and Swiss chard provide fiber, magnesium, and chlorophyll—all great for liver support and internal cleansing.
- **Lemon juice**, especially when added to your morning pink salt flush, enhances digestion, stimulates the liver, and helps alkalize your system.
- **Garlic and onions** are rich in natural detoxifiers and sulfur compounds. They support immune function and help break down toxins in the liver.
- **Coconut oil and coconut milk** contain healthy fats (MCTs) that can fuel your brain and support fat-burning when used in moderation.
- **Apples** are high in fiber and natural pectin, which helps bind and remove toxins from the digestive tract. They're a perfect snack with a pinch of pink salt and a tablespoon of nut butter.
- **Cucumbers** are naturally hydrating, alkaline, and rich in silica. Add them to infused water or eat them raw with hummus and pink salt.
- **Green tea or matcha** helps burn fat, reduce hunger, and deliver antioxidants. Aim for one or two cups daily between meals for a gentle metabolic lift.
- **Sweet potatoes** offer slow-digesting carbs and beta-carotene. They help prevent blood sugar crashes and keep you full longer.
- **Turmeric,** a powerful anti-inflammatory root, supports liver detoxification and joint health. Add it to golden milk, soups, or roasted veggies.
- **Chia and flax seeds** are loaded with omega-3s, fiber, and plant protein. They help with digestion, reduce inflammation, and keep you feeling satisfied.

✅ What You Don't Need

You don't need expensive powders, trendy detox teas, or exotic superfoods that are hard to pronounce or find. Everything listed above is affordable, accessible, and truly functional.

Focus on whole, natural ingredients. Choose foods that love your body back. And remember, the most powerful combination is **pink salt + water + real food.**

Exercise and Mindful Eating Pairings

The Pink Salt Trick Diet is more than a way of eating—it's a lifestyle of balance, nourishment, and intention. While food and hydration lay the foundation, adding gentle movement and mindful eating habits can take your transformation to the next level.

This section guides you on how to pair exercise and meals for better fat burning, digestion, energy, and body awareness, without exhausting your body or triggering burnout.

🏃 Why Exercise Matters in the Pink Salt Lifestyle

Exercise doesn't need to be intense or time-consuming. In fact, overtraining while detoxing can backfire. The right type of movement enhances:

- Lymphatic flow and detoxification
- Insulin sensitivity and fat metabolism
- Digestion and regular elimination
- Mood, sleep, and hormonal balance

Combined with mineral support from pink salt and proper hydration, even 20–30 minutes of intentional movement each day can accelerate results and reduce cravings.

🔄 Best Types of Exercise to Pair With the Diet

1. Morning Walks or Light Cardio

Walking after your Pink Salt Flush stimulates the lymphatic system and jumpstarts fat burning. Just 20–30 minutes is enough to support circulation and mindset.

2. Yoga or Gentle Stretching

Perfect for days when you're cleansing or recalibrating. These practices calm cortisol levels and improve digestion by reducing internal stress.

3. Strength Training

Doing light resistance training 2–3 times a week helps preserve lean muscle during weight loss. Try bodyweight squats, lunges, or light dumbbells after lunch or early evening.

4. Rebounding or Dance

These playful activities move lymph and elevate your mood while supporting natural detox. Great after a nutrient-rich breakfast or smoothie.

5. Evening Walks

A calm walk after dinner helps with blood sugar balance, digestion, and stress relief before bed.

🍽 Mindful Eating for Metabolic Alignment

Mindful eating is the perfect partner to movement. When you eat with awareness, your body becomes more efficient at digesting, absorbing, and using what you consume. Here's how to get started:

- Eliminate distractions. Turn off your phone, TV, or laptop while eating.
- Eat slowly. Chew each bite thoroughly, savor flavors, and pause between bites.
- Express gratitude. Take a deep breath before meals and reflect on how this food nourishes your body.
- Tune into hunger and fullness. Stop when you're satisfied—not stuffed.
- Honor cravings without guilt. Instead of reacting, pause and ask, "What does my body really need?"

These small shifts reduce overeating, improve digestion, and help you build a positive, lasting relationship with food.

🏃 Timing Your Meals Around Movement

- **Before exercise:** Have a light, easily digestible snack or meal with complex carbs and protein—like oatmeal with nut butter or a smoothie with pink salt and banana.

- **After exercise:** Rehydrate with lemon water or herbal tea, then eat a meal rich in lean protein, healthy fats, and fiber (like a quinoa bowl or veggie stir-fry).
- Avoid high-sodium processed foods after workouts. Your body already received mineral support from pink salt—no need to overload.

💡 Realistic Goals for Real Life

This isn't about perfect routines—it's about showing up for your body consistently.

Start with what feels manageable:

- 10 minutes of morning stretching
- A walk after lunch
- One mindful meal a day without screens

Over time, these become natural rhythms that support your weight loss, reduce stress, and anchor your entire lifestyle.

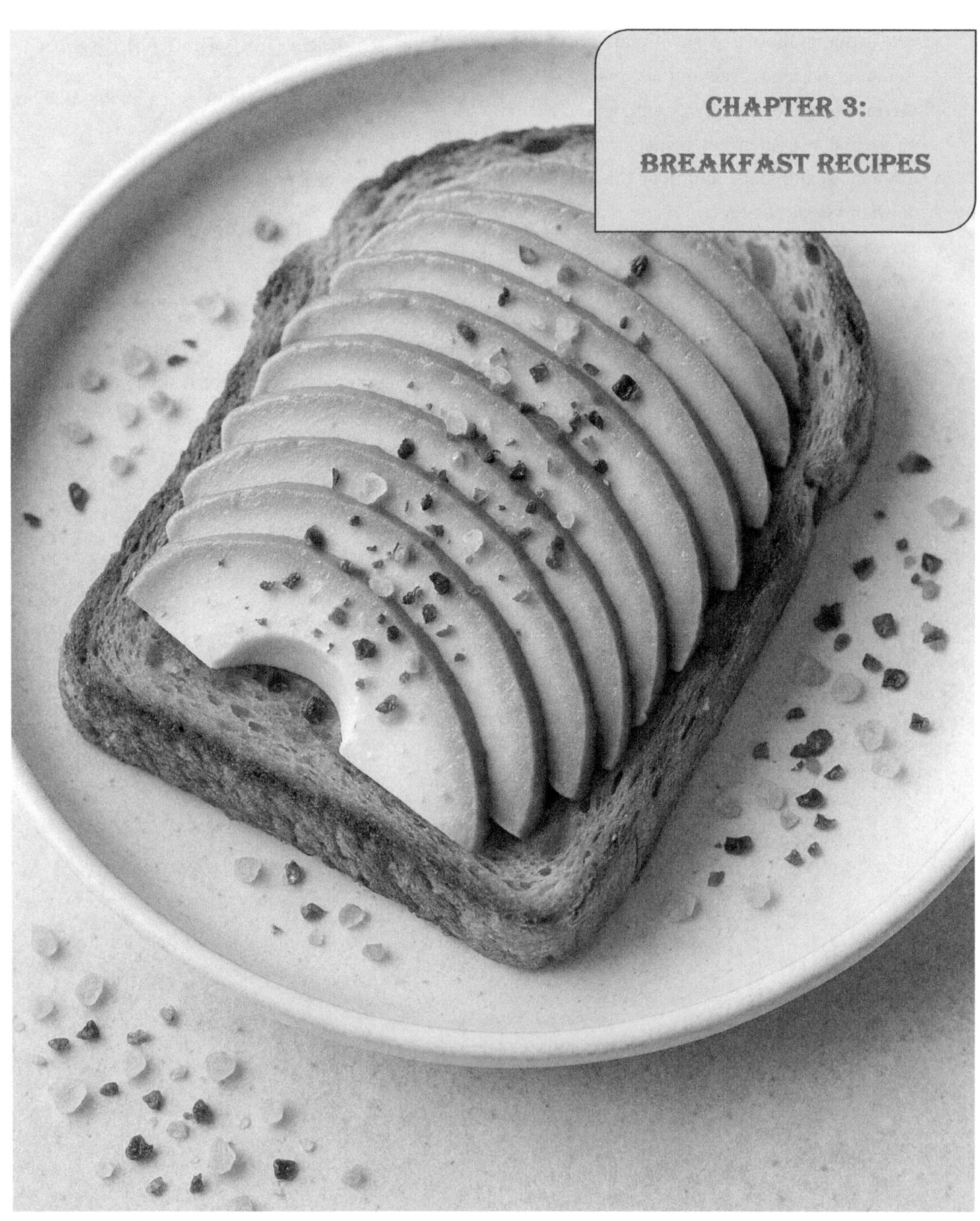

CHAPTER 3:
BREAKFAST RECIPES

48 | The Pink Salt Trick Diet for Weight Loss

Pink Salt Morning Detox Water

Prep Time: 2 mins | Cooking Time: 0 mins | Servings: 1 glass

📝 Ingredients:
- ¼ to ½ teaspoon fine-grain Himalayan pink salt
- 1 cup (8–12 oz) warm filtered water
- Optional: Juice of ½ fresh lemon

👨‍🍳 Instructions:
1. Warm your water until it's comfortably drinkable—not hot or boiling.
2. Add Himalayan pink salt and stir until completely dissolved.
3. (Optional) Squeeze in fresh lemon juice for added detox benefits and flavor.
4. Sip slowly first thing in the morning on an empty stomach.
5. Wait 20–30 minutes before eating or drinking anything else.

🔍 Nutritional Information (per serving):
Calories: 0 | Sodium: 550–1,100 mg | Sugar: 0g | Fat: 0g | Carbs: 0g | Protein: 0g

Avocado Toast with Pink Salt & Chili Flakes

Prep Time: 5 mins | Cooking Time: 2 mins | Servings: 1 slice

📝 Ingredients:
- 1 slice whole grain or sourdough bread
- ½ ripe avocado
- ¼ teaspoon Himalayan pink salt
- Pinch of chili flakes
- 1 teaspoon lemon juice (optional)
- ½ teaspoon extra virgin olive oil (optional)

👨‍🍳 Instructions:
1. Toast the bread to your preferred level of crispiness.
2. In a small bowl, mash the avocado with a fork. Add lemon juice if using.
3. Spread the mashed avocado evenly over the toasted bread.
4. Sprinkle with pink salt and chili flakes.
5. Drizzle with olive oil if desired. Serve immediately.

🔍 Nutritional Information (per serving):
Calories: 210 | Sodium: 300 mg | Sugar: 1g | Fat: 16g | Carbs: 17g | Protein: 4g

Pink Salt Veggie Omelette

Prep Time: 5 mins | Cooking Time: 7 mins | Servings: 1 omelette

📝 Ingredients:
- 2 large eggs
- 1 tablespoon milk or water (for fluffiness)
- ¼ teaspoon Himalayan pink salt
- ¼ cup chopped spinach
- 2 tablespoons chopped bell peppers (any color)
- 2 tablespoons chopped tomatoes
- 1 tablespoon chopped red onion
- Pinch of black pepper and chili flakes (optional)
- 1 teaspoon olive oil or butter

👨‍🍳 Instructions:
1. In a bowl, whisk together eggs, milk or water, pink salt, and black pepper.
2. Heat olive oil or butter in a nonstick skillet over medium heat.
3. Sauté onions, bell peppers, and tomatoes for 2–3 minutes until slightly softened.
4. Add spinach and cook for another 30 seconds.
5. Pour in the egg mixture and swirl to evenly coat the pan.
6. Cook for 2–3 minutes, then gently fold the omelette in half.
7. Cook 1–2 more minutes until fully set. Serve hot.

🔍 Nutritional Information (per serving):
Calories: 220 | Sodium: 430 mg | Sugar: 2g | Fat: 17g | Carbs: 5g | Protein: 12g

Greek Yogurt Parfait with Pink Salted Granola

Prep Time: 5 mins | Cooking Time: 0 mins | Servings: 1 bowl

📝 Ingredients:
- ½ cup plain Greek yogurt
- ¼ cup pink salted granola
- ¼ cup mixed berries (blueberries, strawberries, raspberries)
- 1 teaspoon raw honey or maple syrup (optional)
- Pinch of Himalayan pink salt
- *Note:* Use homemade or store-bought granola seasoned lightly with Himalayan pink salt.

👨‍🍳 Instructions:
1. In a serving bowl or jar, layer half the Greek yogurt.
2. Add a layer of berries and half the granola.
3. Repeat with remaining yogurt, berries, and granola.
4. Drizzle with honey or syrup if using, and sprinkle a tiny pinch of pink salt on top.
5. Serve immediately for crunch, or chill for 10 minutes to slightly soften the granola.

🔍 Nutritional Information (per serving):
Calories: 230 | Sodium: 180 mg | Sugar: 9g | Fat: 7g | Carbs: 27g | Protein: 14g

Chia Pudding with Pink Salted Mango

Prep Time: 5 mins | Cooking Time: 0 mins | Servings: 1 jar

Ingredients:
- 3 tablespoons chia seeds
- ¾ cup unsweetened almond milk (or milk of choice)
- ½ teaspoon vanilla extract
- 1 teaspoon maple syrup or honey (optional)
- ½ cup diced ripe mango
- Pinch of Himalayan pink salt

Instructions:
1. In a jar or bowl, mix chia seeds, almond milk, vanilla, and sweetener (if using).
2. Stir well to prevent clumping, then cover and refrigerate for at least 4 hours or overnight.
3. Just before serving, dice the mango and toss with a pinch of pink salt.
4. Spoon the salted mango over the chilled chia pudding.
5. Serve cold and enjoy!

Nutritional Information (per serving):
Calories: 240 | Sodium: 150 mg | Sugar: 10g | Fat: 11g | Carbs: 27g | Protein: 6g

Almond Butter Pink Salt Smoothie

Prep Time: 3 mins | Cooking Time: 0 mins | Servings: 1 glass

Ingredients:
- 1 ripe banana
- 1 tablespoon almond butter
- ¾ cup unsweetened almond milk
- 1 teaspoon chia seeds
- ¼ teaspoon Himalayan pink salt
- ½ teaspoon cinnamon (optional)
- 4–5 ice cubes

Instructions:
1. Add all ingredients to a blender.
2. Blend on high until smooth and creamy.
3. Taste and adjust pink salt if needed.
4. Pour into a glass and serve immediately.

Nutritional Information (per serving):
Calories: 210 | Sodium: 270 mg | Sugar: 10g | Fat: 10g | Carbs: 25g | Protein: 5g

Protein Pancakes with Pink Salted Berries

Prep Time: 7 mins ⏱ | Cooking Time: 10 mins 🔥 | Servings: 2 pancakes 🍽

📝 Ingredients:
- 1 ripe banana 🍌
- 2 large eggs 🥚
- 2 tablespoons protein powder (vanilla or unflavored) 💪
- ¼ teaspoon baking powder 🧁
- ¼ teaspoon Himalayan pink salt 🧂
- ¼ teaspoon cinnamon (optional) 🥮
- ½ cup mixed berries (blueberries, strawberries, raspberries) 🫐
- ½ teaspoon raw honey or maple syrup (optional) 🍯
- Nonstick spray or ½ teaspoon coconut oil for cooking 🥥

👨‍🍳 Instructions:
1. In a bowl, mash the banana and whisk in eggs until well combined.
2. Add protein powder, baking powder, cinnamon (if using), and pink salt. Mix until smooth.
3. Heat a nonstick skillet over medium heat and grease lightly.
4. Pour batter to form two pancakes. Cook for 2–3 minutes on each side until golden and set.
5. While pancakes cook, lightly mash the berries in a bowl and sprinkle with a pinch of pink salt.
6. Serve pancakes topped with pink salted berries and a drizzle of honey or syrup if desired.

🔍 Nutritional Information (per serving):
Calories: 280 🔥 | Sodium: 320 mg 🧂 | Sugar: 9g 🔍 | Fat: 10g 🧈 | Carbs: 25g 🍞 | Protein: 18g 🔍

Overnight Oats with Himalayan Sea Salt & Figs

Prep Time: 5 mins ⏱ | Cooking Time: 0 mins ⊘ | Servings: 1 jar ☐

📝 Ingredients:
- ½ cup rolled oats 🌾
- ½ cup unsweetened almond milk (or milk of choice) 🥛
- 1 tablespoon chia seeds 🌱
- ¼ teaspoon Himalayan pink salt 🧂
- ½ teaspoon vanilla extract 🌸
- 1 teaspoon maple syrup or honey (optional) 🍯
- 2 dried or fresh figs, sliced 🍑
- 1 tablespoon chopped walnuts or pecans (optional) 🥮

👨‍🍳 Instructions:
1. In a mason jar or bowl, combine oats, almond milk, chia seeds, vanilla, and pink salt.
2. Stir well to combine and ensure chia seeds don't clump.
3. Seal and refrigerate overnight or at least 4 hours.
4. Before serving, top with sliced figs and nuts.
5. Drizzle with maple syrup or honey if desired. Enjoy cold or at room temperature.

🔍 Nutritional Information (per serving):
Calories: 310 🔥 | Sodium: 260 mg 🧂 | Sugar: 12g 🔍 | Fat: 11g 🧈 | Carbs: 40g 🍞 | Protein: 8g 🔍

Breakfast Quinoa Bowl with Banana and Pink Salt

Prep Time: 5 mins | Cooking Time: 15 mins | Servings: 1 bowl

📝 Ingredients:
- ½ cup cooked quinoa
- ½ cup unsweetened almond milk (or milk of choice)
- 1 ripe banana, sliced
- ¼ teaspoon Himalayan pink salt
- ¼ teaspoon cinnamon
- 1 teaspoon chia seeds
- 1 teaspoon maple syrup or honey (optional)
- 1 tablespoon chopped walnuts or almonds (optional)

👨‍🍳 Instructions:
1. In a small saucepan, combine cooked quinoa and almond milk over medium heat.
2. Stir in cinnamon and pink salt. Simmer for 5–7 minutes until warm and creamy.
3. Transfer to a bowl and top with sliced banana.
4. Sprinkle with chia seeds and nuts if using.
5. Drizzle with honey or maple syrup for added sweetness, if desired. Serve warm.

🔍 Nutritional Information (per serving):
Calories: 290 | Sodium: 240 mg | Sugar: 10g | Fat: 9g | Carbs: 38g | Protein: 8g

Tofu Scramble with Pink Salt

Prep Time: 5 mins | Cooking Time: 10 mins | Servings: 1 plate

📝 Ingredients:
- ½ block (about 200g) firm tofu, drained and crumbled
- ¼ teaspoon Himalayan pink salt
- ¼ teaspoon turmeric powder (for color and health benefits)
- ¼ teaspoon black pepper or chili flakes
- 1 tablespoon olive oil or avocado oil
- 2 tablespoons chopped onions
- 2 tablespoons chopped bell peppers
- ¼ cup spinach or kale, chopped
- Optional: Nutritional yeast or a squeeze of lemon for added flavor

👨‍🍳 Instructions:
1. Heat oil in a nonstick skillet over medium heat.
2. Add onions and bell peppers. Sauté for 2–3 minutes until softened.
3. Stir in crumbled tofu, turmeric, pink salt, and pepper. Mix well to coat evenly.
4. Cook for 5–7 minutes, stirring occasionally, until slightly golden.
5. Add spinach or kale and cook for another minute until wilted.
6. Serve warm. Add lemon juice or nutritional yeast if desired.

🔍 Nutritional Information (per serving):
Calories: 220 | Sodium: 320 mg | Sugar: 2g | Fat: 14g | Carbs: 8g | Protein: 14g

Cinnamon-Spiced Apple Bake with Pink Salt

Prep Time: 10 mins | Cooking Time: 25 mins | Servings: 2 bowls

Ingredients:
- 2 medium apples, cored and sliced thin
- 1 teaspoon coconut oil or melted butter
- ½ teaspoon ground cinnamon
- ¼ teaspoon Himalayan pink salt
- 1 teaspoon maple syrup or honey (optional)
- 1 tablespoon chopped walnuts or pecans (optional)
- ½ teaspoon vanilla extract
- Juice of ¼ lemon

Instructions:
1. Preheat oven to 350°F (175°C).
2. In a mixing bowl, toss apple slices with coconut oil, cinnamon, pink salt, lemon juice, and vanilla.
3. Spread mixture evenly in a small baking dish.
4. Drizzle with maple syrup or honey if using, and sprinkle with nuts.
5. Bake uncovered for 20–25 minutes, or until apples are soft and caramelized.
6. Let cool slightly before serving. Enjoy warm for breakfast or dessert.

Nutritional Information (per serving):
Calories: 160 | Sodium: 180 mg | Sugar: 12g | Fat: 7g | Carbs: 22g | Protein: 1g

Blueberry Protein Shake with Pink Salt

Prep Time: 3 mins | Cooking Time: 0 mins | Servings: 1 glass

Ingredients:
- ½ cup frozen blueberries
- 1 scoop vanilla or unflavored protein powder
- ¾ cup unsweetened almond milk (or milk of choice)
- 1 tablespoon chia seeds or flaxseeds
- ¼ teaspoon Himalayan pink salt
- ½ teaspoon cinnamon (optional)
- 1–2 ice cubes

Instructions:
1. Add all ingredients to a high-speed blender.
2. Blend until smooth and creamy.
3. Taste and adjust pink salt to your liking.
4. Pour into a glass and enjoy immediately.

Nutritional Information (per serving):
Calories: 220 | Sodium: 280 mg | Sugar: 6g | Fat: 8g | Carbs: 15g | Protein: 20g

Pink Salt & Turmeric Coconut Milk

Prep Time: 3 mins | Cooking Time: 5 mins | Servings: 1 cup

Ingredients:
- 1 cup unsweetened coconut milk
- ¼ teaspoon ground turmeric
- ¼ teaspoon Himalayan pink salt
- ¼ teaspoon ground cinnamon (optional)
- Pinch of black pepper (to enhance turmeric absorption)
- 1 teaspoon raw honey or maple syrup (optional)

Instructions:
1. In a small saucepan, combine coconut milk, turmeric, pink salt, cinnamon (if using), and black pepper.
2. Heat gently over medium-low heat, stirring continuously for 4–5 minutes.
3. Do not boil—just warm until steamy and well blended.
4. Remove from heat and stir in honey or syrup if desired.
5. Pour into a mug and sip slowly, preferably in the evening or morning.

Nutritional Information (per serving):
Calories: 120 | Sodium: 250 mg | Sugar: 4g | Fat: 9g | Carbs: 7g | Protein: 1g

Gluten-Free Breakfast Muffins with a Pink Salt Twist

Prep Time: 10 mins | Cooking Time: 20 mins | Servings: 6 muffins

Ingredients:
- 1 cup almond flour
- ¼ cup gluten-free rolled oats
- 2 large eggs
- 1 ripe banana, mashed
- 2 tablespoons maple syrup or honey
- ¼ cup unsweetened almond milk
- 1 teaspoon baking powder
- ¼ teaspoon ground cinnamon
- ¼ teaspoon Himalayan pink salt
- ¼ cup blueberries or chopped apples (optional)

Instructions:
1. Preheat oven to 350°F (175°C) and line a muffin tin with paper liners.
2. In a large bowl, whisk together eggs, mashed banana, almond milk, and sweetener.
3. Add almond flour, oats, baking powder, cinnamon, and pink salt. Mix well to combine.
4. Fold in fruit if using.
5. Divide batter evenly into 6 muffin cups.
6. Bake for 18–20 minutes or until a toothpick comes out clean.
7. Let cool slightly before serving. Perfect for grab-and-go mornings!

Nutritional Information (per muffin):
Calories: 160 | Sodium: 180 mg | Sugar: 6g | Fat: 9g | Carbs: 14g | Protein: 5g

Zucchini Hash with Poached Egg and Pink Salt

Prep Time: 7 mins | Cooking Time: 10 mins | Servings: 1 plate

Ingredients:
- 1 medium zucchini, grated or finely chopped
- ¼ cup chopped bell peppers
- 2 tablespoons chopped red onion
- 1 teaspoon olive oil
- 1 large egg
- ¼ teaspoon Himalayan pink salt
- Pinch of black pepper
- Optional: fresh herbs (parsley or chives) for garnish

Instructions:
1. Heat olive oil in a skillet over medium heat.
2. Add onion and bell pepper; sauté for 2–3 minutes.
3. Stir in zucchini, season with pink salt and pepper, and cook for 4–5 minutes until tender and lightly golden.
4. Meanwhile, poach the egg: bring a small pot of water to a gentle simmer, crack in the egg, and cook for 3–4 minutes until the white is set.
5. Plate the zucchini hash, top with the poached egg, and sprinkle with a touch more pink salt.
6. Garnish with herbs if desired. Serve immediately.

Nutritional Information (per serving):
Calories: 190 | Sodium: 300 mg | Sugar: 5g | Fat: 12g | Carbs: 9g | Protein: 9g

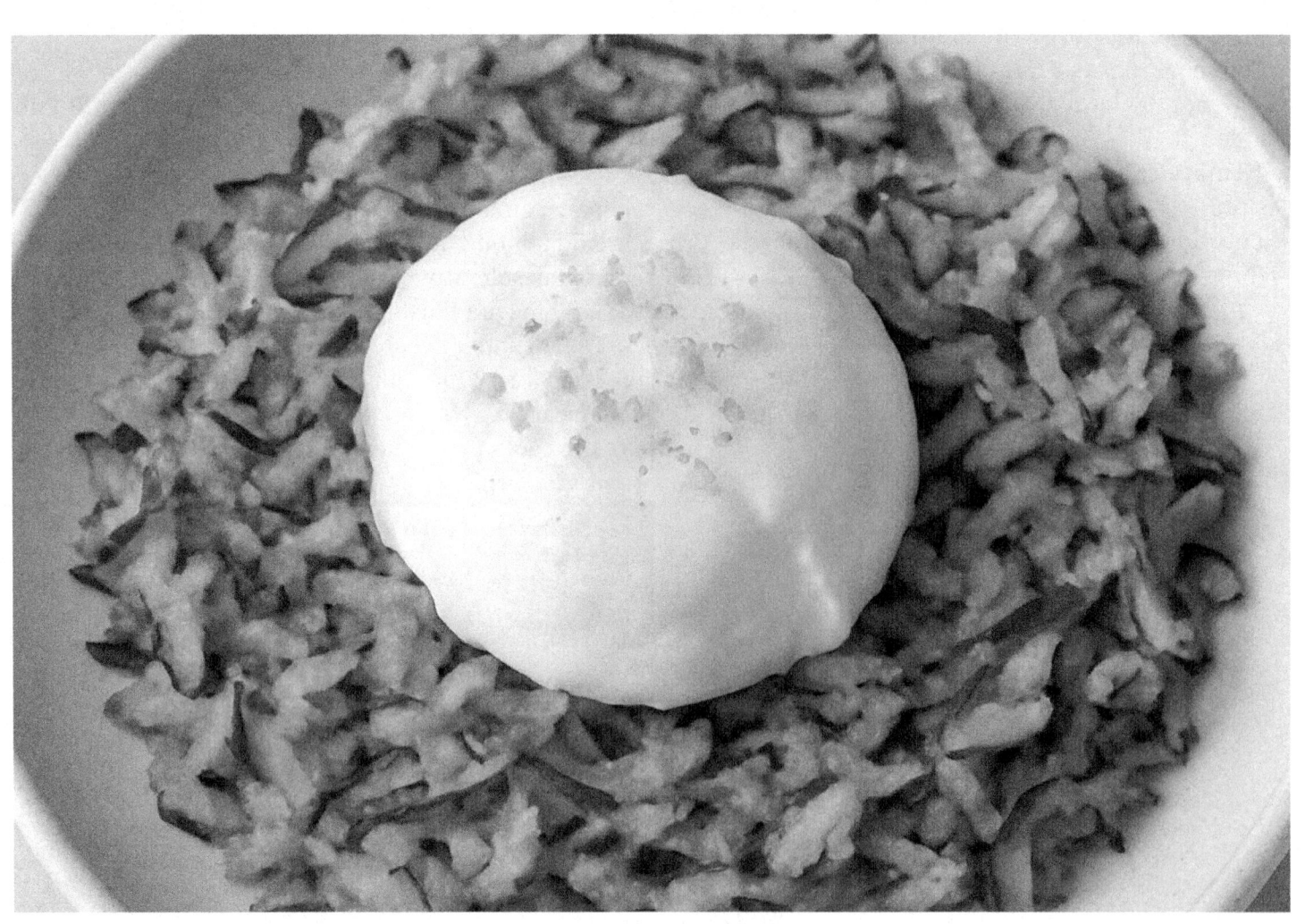

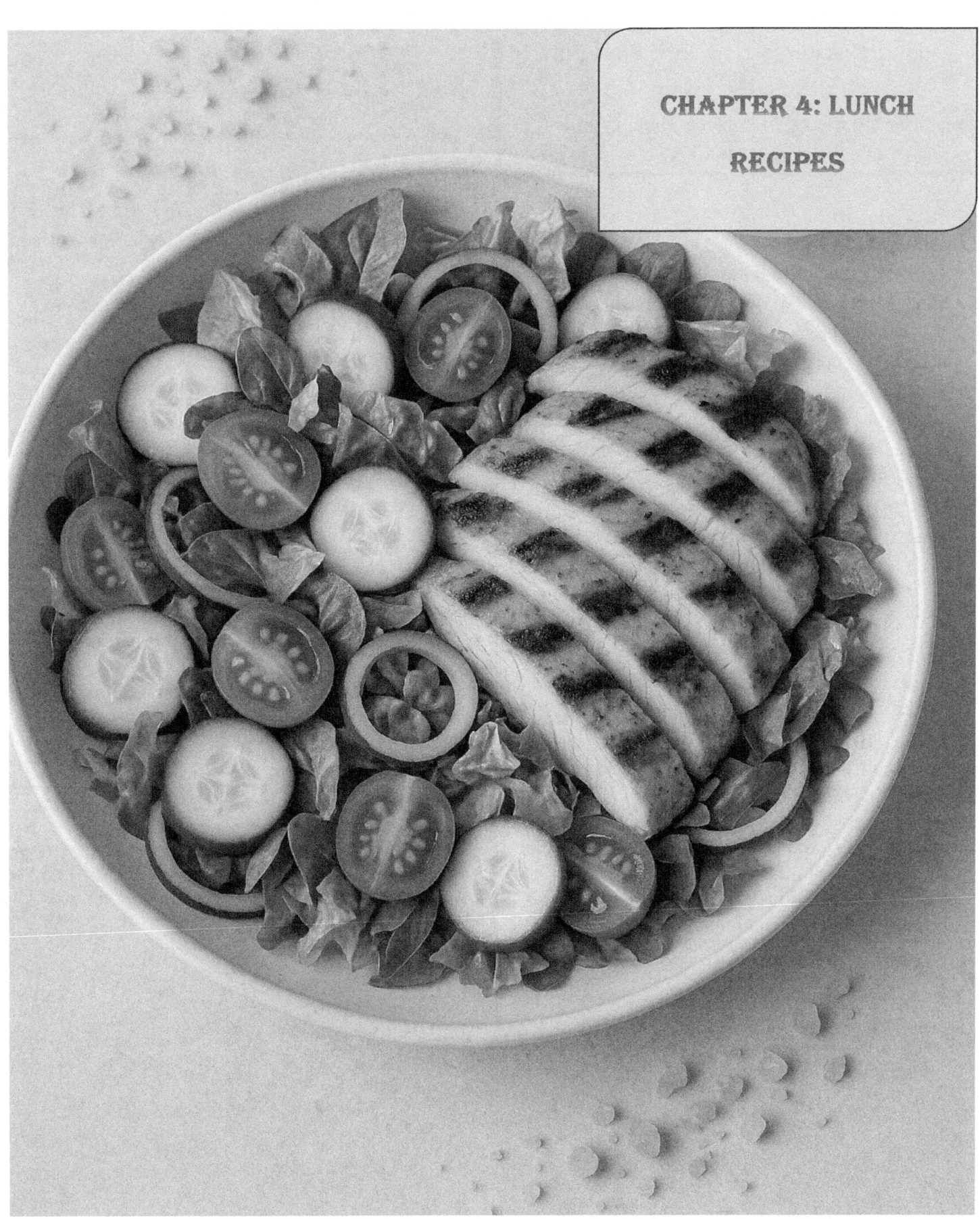

CHAPTER 4: LUNCH RECIPES

Grilled Chicken Salad with Pink Salt Citrus Dressing

Prep Time: 10 mins ⏲ | Cooking Time: 15 mins 🔥 | Servings: 1 bowl 🍽

📝 Ingredients:
For the Salad:
- 1 grilled chicken breast, sliced 🍗
- 1 cup mixed greens (spinach, arugula, romaine) 🥬
- ¼ cup cherry tomatoes, halved 🍅
- ¼ cucumber, sliced 🥒
- 1 tablespoon red onion, thinly sliced 🧅
- 1 tablespoon toasted sunflower seeds or sliced almonds 🌻

For the Pink Salt Citrus Dressing:
- 1 tablespoon olive oil 🫒
- 1 tablespoon fresh lemon juice 🍋
- ½ teaspoon Dijon mustard
- ¼ teaspoon Himalayan pink salt 🧂
- Pinch of black pepper 🌶
- ½ teaspoon honey or maple syrup (optional) 🍯

👨‍🍳 Instructions:
1. In a small bowl, whisk together all the dressing ingredients until well emulsified.
2. In a large serving bowl, layer the greens, tomatoes, cucumber, onion, and grilled chicken.
3. Drizzle with the pink salt citrus dressing.
4. Sprinkle with sunflower seeds or almonds.
5. Toss gently and serve immediately.

🔍 Nutritional Information (per serving):
Calories: 310 🔥 | Sodium: 320 mg 🧂 | Sugar: 4g 🍭 | Fat: 18g 🥓 | Carbs: 9g 🍞 | Protein: 28g 🍖

Pink Salt Tuna Lettuce Wraps

Prep Time: 8 mins ⏲ | Cooking Time: 0 mins 🚫 | Servings: 2 wraps 🌮

📝 Ingredients:
- 1 (5 oz) can tuna in water, drained 🐟
- 1 tablespoon plain Greek yogurt or avocado mayo 🥑
- 1 teaspoon Dijon mustard
- ¼ teaspoon Himalayan pink salt 🧂
- 1 tablespoon chopped celery 🥬
- 1 tablespoon finely chopped red onion 🧅
- 1 teaspoon lemon juice 🍋
- 2 large romaine or butter lettuce leaves 🥬
- Optional: sliced cherry tomatoes, avocado, or cucumber for topping 🍅🥒

👨‍🍳 Instructions:
1. In a bowl, mix tuna, Greek yogurt (or mayo), mustard, pink salt, celery, onion, and lemon juice until well combined.
2. Spoon the tuna mixture into the center of each lettuce leaf.
3. Top with your favorite optional add-ons like avocado or tomatoes.
4. Fold gently and serve immediately, or chill for 10–15 minutes before eating.

🔍 Nutritional Information (per serving – 2 wraps):
Calories: 210 🔥 | Sodium: 290 mg 🧂 | Sugar: 2g 🍭 | Fat: 9g 🥓 | Carbs: 4g 🍞 | Protein: 27g 🍖

Roasted Veggie & Quinoa Bowl with Pink Salt

Prep Time: 10 mins | Cooking Time: 25 mins | Servings: 1 bowl

📝 Ingredients:
- ½ cup cooked quinoa
- ½ cup chopped sweet potatoes
- ¼ cup chopped zucchini
- ¼ cup chopped bell peppers
- ¼ cup broccoli florets
- 1 tablespoon olive oil
- ¼ teaspoon Himalayan pink salt
- ¼ teaspoon black pepper
- 1 tablespoon tahini or hummus (optional)
- Fresh lemon juice for garnish

👨‍🍳 Instructions:
1. Preheat oven to 400°F (200°C).
2. Toss sweet potatoes, zucchini, bell peppers, and broccoli with olive oil, pink salt, and black pepper.
3. Spread veggies on a baking sheet and roast for 20–25 minutes, flipping halfway through.
4. In a bowl, layer the cooked quinoa with roasted vegetables.
5. Top with tahini or hummus if using, and a squeeze of fresh lemon juice.
6. Serve warm or at room temperature.

🔍 Nutritional Information (per serving):
Calories: 320 | Sodium: 270 mg | Sugar: 6g | Fat: 13g | Carbs: 38g | Protein: 10g

---

Chickpea Salad with Cucumber, Dill & Pink Salt

Prep Time: 10 mins | Cooking Time: 0 mins | Servings: 1 bowl

📝 Ingredients:
- ½ cup canned chickpeas, rinsed and drained
- ¼ cup diced cucumber
- 1 tablespoon chopped fresh dill
- 1 tablespoon chopped red onion
- 1 tablespoon olive oil
- 1 teaspoon fresh lemon juice
- ¼ teaspoon Himalayan pink salt
- Pinch of black pepper
- Optional: crumbled feta or diced avocado

👨‍🍳 Instructions:
1. In a medium bowl, combine chickpeas, cucumber, dill, and red onion.
2. Drizzle with olive oil and lemon juice.
3. Season with pink salt and black pepper.
4. Toss everything gently until well combined.
5. Top with optional feta or avocado if desired. Serve chilled or at room temperature.

🔍 Nutritional Information (per serving):
Calories: 220 | Sodium: 290 mg | Sugar: 3g | Fat: 11g | Carbs: 22g | Protein: 6g

Zesty Pink Salt Shrimp Stir-Fry

Prep Time: 10 mins | Cooking Time: 10 mins | Servings: 1 plate

Ingredients:
- ½ lb (about 225g) raw shrimp, peeled and deveined
- 1 tablespoon olive oil or sesame oil
- 1 clove garlic, minced
- 1 teaspoon fresh ginger, grated
- ¼ cup sliced bell peppers
- ¼ cup snap peas or broccoli florets
- 1 tablespoon fresh lemon or lime juice
- ¼ teaspoon Himalayan pink salt
- Pinch of red pepper flakes (optional)
- Optional garnish: chopped green onions or sesame seeds

Instructions:
1. Heat oil in a skillet or wok over medium-high heat.
2. Add garlic and ginger, stir for 30 seconds until fragrant.
3. Toss in shrimp and cook for 2–3 minutes per side until pink and opaque.
4. Add bell peppers and snap peas; stir-fry for 2–3 more minutes.
5. Drizzle with lemon or lime juice and season with pink salt and red pepper flakes.
6. Garnish with green onions or sesame seeds if desired. Serve hot.

Nutritional Information (per serving):
Calories: 280 | Sodium: 330 mg | Sugar: 2g | Fat: 14g | Carbs: 6g | Protein: 32g

Lentil Soup with Pink Salt and Thyme

Prep Time: 10 mins | Cooking Time: 30 mins | Servings: 2 bowls

Ingredients:
- ½ cup dried lentils (green or brown), rinsed
- 1 tablespoon olive oil
- ½ small onion, chopped
- 1 small carrot, diced
- 1 celery stalk, diced
- 1 garlic clove, minced
- ½ teaspoon dried thyme
- ¼ teaspoon Himalayan pink salt
- ⅛ teaspoon black pepper
- 2 cups vegetable broth or water
- Juice of ¼ lemon (optional)

Instructions:
1. In a pot, heat olive oil over medium heat. Add onion, carrot, and celery. Sauté for 5–6 minutes until softened.
2. Add garlic and thyme; cook for 1 minute.
3. Stir in lentils, pink salt, pepper, and broth. Bring to a boil.
4. Reduce heat, cover, and simmer for 25–30 minutes until lentils are tender.
5. Taste and adjust seasoning. Stir in lemon juice if using.
6. Serve warm with fresh herbs or crusty gluten-free bread, if desired.

Nutritional Information (per serving):
Calories: 210 | Sodium: 310 mg | Sugar: 4g | Fat: 7g | Carbs: 28g | Protein: 10g

Pink Salted Kale and Avocado Rice Bowl

Prep Time: 10 mins | Cooking Time: 15 mins | Servings: 1 bowl

📝 Ingredients:
- ½ cup cooked brown rice or quinoa
- 1 cup chopped kale, stems removed
- ½ avocado, sliced
- 1 teaspoon olive oil
- 1 teaspoon lemon juice
- ¼ teaspoon Himalayan pink salt
- Pinch of black pepper
- 1 tablespoon toasted pumpkin seeds (optional)
- 1 soft-boiled or poached egg (optional)

👨‍🍳 Instructions:
1. In a skillet over medium heat, warm olive oil and sauté chopped kale for 3–4 minutes until wilted.
2. Season kale with pink salt, pepper, and lemon juice. Remove from heat.
3. In a bowl, layer the cooked rice or quinoa as the base.
4. Add sautéed kale and top with sliced avocado.
5. Sprinkle with pumpkin seeds and add egg if using.
6. Serve warm or room temperature with an extra pinch of pink salt if desired.

🔍 Nutritional Information (per serving):
Calories: 310 | Sodium: 280 mg | Sugar: 2g | Fat: 18g | Carbs: 28g | Protein: 9g

Baked Falafel with Pink Salt & Tahini Sauce

Prep Time: 15 mins | Cooking Time: 25 mins | Servings: 2 portions

📝 Ingredients:
For the Falafel:
- 1 cup canned chickpeas, rinsed and drained
- 2 tablespoons chopped fresh parsley
- 1 clove garlic, minced
- 2 tablespoons chopped onion
- 1 tablespoon oat flour or almond flour
- ½ teaspoon ground cumin
- ¼ teaspoon ground coriander
- ¼ teaspoon Himalayan pink salt
- 1 tablespoon olive oil (for brushing)

For the Tahini Sauce:
- 1 tablespoon tahini
- 1 tablespoon lemon juice
- 1 tablespoon water
- ⅛ teaspoon Himalayan pink salt
- Pinch of garlic powder (optional)

👨‍🍳 Instructions:
1. Preheat oven to 375°F (190°C) and line a baking sheet with parchment paper.
2. In a food processor, combine chickpeas, parsley, garlic, onion, flour, cumin, coriander, and pink salt. Pulse until a coarse mixture forms.
3. Shape into 6 small balls or patties and place on the baking sheet.
4. Brush lightly with olive oil.
5. Bake for 20–25 minutes, flipping halfway, until golden and crisp on the outside.
6. Meanwhile, whisk together all tahini sauce ingredients in a small bowl until smooth. Serve falafel warm with sauce on the side or drizzled on top.

🔍 Nutritional Information (per serving – 3 falafel + sauce):
Calories: 280 | Sodium: 290 mg | Sugar: 2g | Fat: 15g | Carbs: 24g | Protein: 9g

Asian Slaw with Pink Salt Sesame Dressing

Prep Time: 10 mins | Cooking Time: 0 mins | Servings: 1 bowl

Ingredients:

For the Slaw:
- 1 cup shredded green cabbage
- ½ cup shredded purple cabbage
- ¼ cup shredded carrots
- 2 tablespoons sliced green onions
- 1 tablespoon chopped cilantro (optional)

For the Pink Salt Sesame Dressing:
- 1 tablespoon sesame oil
- 1 teaspoon rice vinegar
- ½ teaspoon low-sodium soy sauce or tamari
- ¼ teaspoon Himalayan pink salt
- ½ teaspoon maple syrup or honey
- ½ teaspoon grated fresh ginger
- Optional: pinch of red pepper flakes

Instructions:

1. In a large mixing bowl, combine all slaw ingredients and toss gently.
2. In a small bowl, whisk together all dressing ingredients until smooth and well blended.
3. Pour dressing over the slaw and toss until evenly coated.
4. Let sit for 5–10 minutes to allow flavors to meld.
5. Serve chilled or at room temperature.

Nutritional Information (per serving):

Calories: 170 | Sodium: 260 mg | Sugar: 5g | Fat: 12g | Carbs: 13g | Protein: 2g

---

Pink Salt Marinated Grilled Tofu Bowl

Prep Time: 15 mins | Cooking Time: 15 mins | Servings: 1 bowl

Ingredients:

For the Tofu Marinade:
- ½ block firm tofu (about 150g), pressed and sliced into cubes
- 1 tablespoon olive oil
- 1 tablespoon low-sodium soy sauce or tamari
- ¼ teaspoon Himalayan pink salt
- 1 teaspoon rice vinegar
- ½ teaspoon maple syrup or honey
- ½ teaspoon grated fresh ginger
- 1 clove garlic, minced

For the Bowl:
- ½ cup cooked brown rice or quinoa
- ½ cup steamed or sautéed broccoli
- ¼ cup shredded carrots
- ¼ avocado, sliced
- 1 tablespoon chopped green onions or sesame seeds (optional)

Instructions:

1. In a bowl, whisk together all marinade ingredients.
2. Add tofu cubes and let marinate for at least 15 minutes (up to overnight).
3. Heat a grill pan or skillet over medium heat. Grill tofu pieces for 3–4 minutes on each side until golden.
4. In a serving bowl, layer cooked rice or quinoa with broccoli, carrots, and avocado.
5. Top with grilled tofu and sprinkle with optional garnishes.
6. Serve warm with an extra pinch of pink salt if desired.

Nutritional Information (per serving):

Calories: 360 | Sodium: 310 mg | Sugar: 5g | Fat: 20g | Carbs: 28g | Protein: 16g

Mushroom and Pink Salt Risotto

Prep Time: 10 mins | Cooking Time: 25 mins | Servings: 1 bowl

Ingredients:
- ½ cup arborio rice
- 1 cup low-sodium vegetable broth (warmed)
- ½ cup sliced mushrooms (cremini or button)
- 1 tablespoon olive oil or unsalted butter
- 1 tablespoon chopped onion
- 1 clove garlic, minced
- ¼ teaspoon Himalayan pink salt
- ⅛ teaspoon black pepper
- 1 tablespoon grated Parmesan cheese (optional)
- 1 teaspoon chopped fresh parsley for garnish

Instructions:
1. Heat olive oil or butter in a saucepan over medium heat. Add onions and cook until translucent, about 2–3 minutes.
2. Add garlic and mushrooms. Cook for 4–5 minutes until mushrooms are tender.
3. Stir in arborio rice and toast for 1–2 minutes.
4. Begin adding the warm broth, ¼ cup at a time, stirring constantly until liquid is absorbed before adding more.
5. Continue this process for 20–25 minutes, or until rice is creamy and tender.
6. Season with pink salt and black pepper.
7. Stir in Parmesan (if using) and garnish with parsley. Serve warm.

Nutritional Information (per serving):
Calories: 330 | Sodium: 320 mg | Sugar: 3g | Fat: 14g | Carbs: 42g | Protein: 7g

Turmeric Chicken and Pink Salt Couscous

Prep Time: 10 mins | Cooking Time: 20 mins | Servings: 1 plate

Ingredients:
For the Chicken:
- 1 small chicken breast, cut into strips
- ½ teaspoon ground turmeric
- ¼ teaspoon Himalayan pink salt
- ¼ teaspoon black pepper
- 1 tablespoon olive oil
- ½ teaspoon garlic powder

For the Couscous:
- ½ cup whole wheat or regular couscous
- ½ cup boiling water
- ¼ teaspoon Himalayan pink salt
- 1 teaspoon olive oil
- 1 tablespoon chopped parsley (optional)
- Juice of ¼ lemon

Instructions:
1. In a bowl, toss chicken strips with turmeric, pink salt, pepper, garlic powder, and olive oil.
2. Heat a skillet over medium heat. Cook chicken for 4–5 minutes per side until golden and cooked through.
3. Meanwhile, in a bowl, combine couscous, pink salt, olive oil, and boiling water. Cover and let sit for 5 minutes, then fluff with a fork.
4. Stir in lemon juice and parsley.
5. Serve turmeric chicken over couscous. Garnish with extra herbs or lemon wedges if desired.

Nutritional Information (per serving):
Calories: 370 | Sodium: 350 mg | Sugar: 1g | Fat: 17g | Carbs: 28g | Protein: 28g

Stuffed Bell Peppers with Pink Salt Quinoa Mix

Prep Time: 15 mins ⏱ | Cooking Time: 30 mins 🔥 | Servings: 2 stuffed peppers 🍽

📝 Ingredients:
- 2 large bell peppers, tops sliced off and seeds removed 🫑
- ½ cup cooked quinoa 🌿
- ¼ cup canned black beans, rinsed and drained ♥
- ¼ cup diced tomatoes 🍅
- 2 tablespoons chopped onion 🧅
- 1 tablespoon chopped cilantro (optional) 🌿
- ½ teaspoon cumin 🌱
- ¼ teaspoon smoked paprika 🌶
- ¼ teaspoon Himalayan pink salt 🧂
- 1 teaspoon olive oil 🫒
- Optional: shredded cheese for topping 🧀

👨‍🍳 Instructions:
1. Preheat oven to 375°F (190°C).
2. In a skillet, heat olive oil over medium heat. Sauté onions for 2–3 minutes until soft.
3. Add quinoa, black beans, tomatoes, cilantro, and spices. Stir well and cook for 2–3 minutes.
4. Stuff the bell peppers with the quinoa mixture and place in a baking dish.
5. Cover with foil and bake for 25–30 minutes until peppers are tender.
6. Uncover in the last 5 minutes and top with cheese if using. Serve warm.

🔍 Nutritional Information (per serving – 1 stuffed pepper):
Calories: 230 🔥 | Sodium: 300 mg 🧂 | Sugar: 6g 🔍 | Fat: 8g 🧈 | Carbs: 28g 🍞 | Protein: 9g 🔍

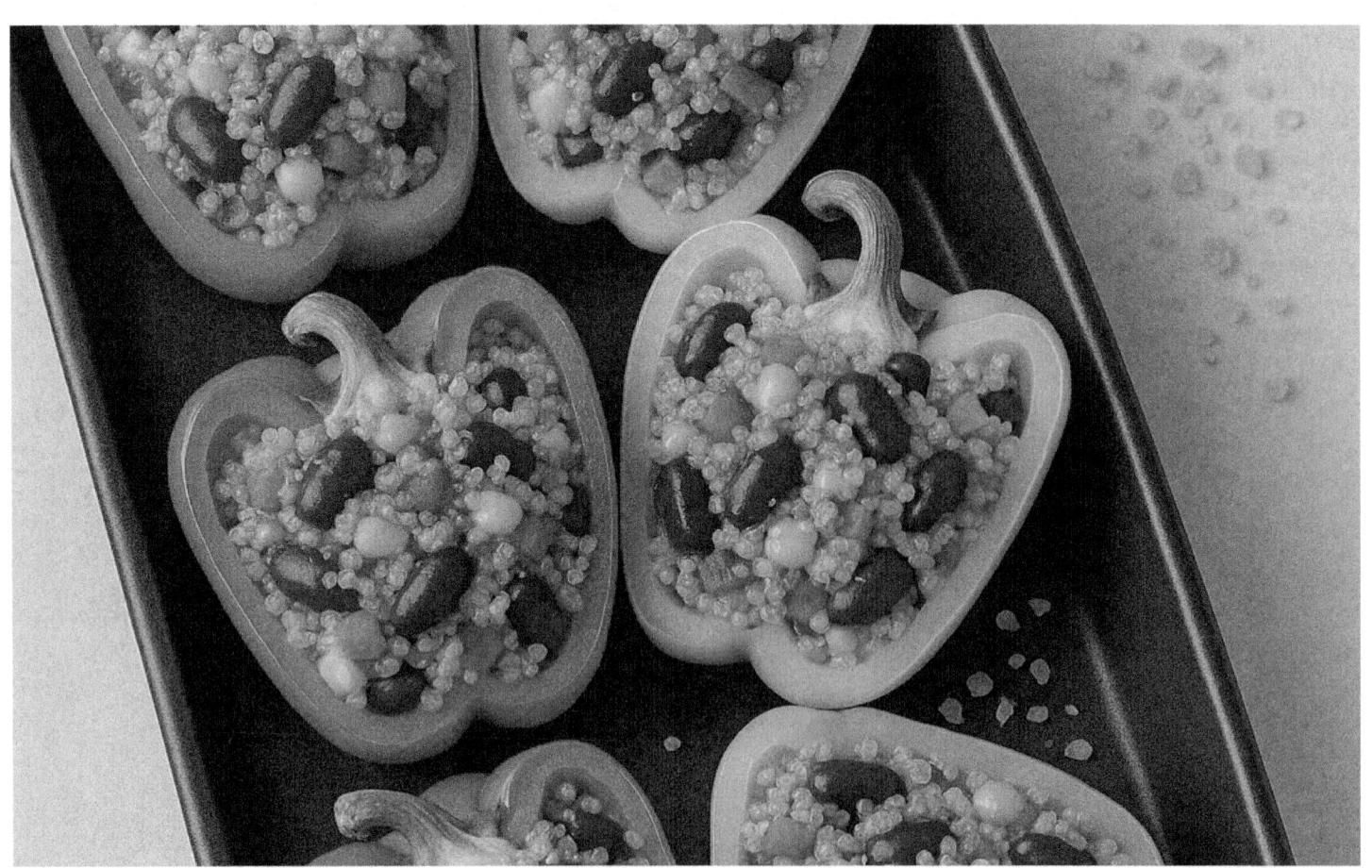

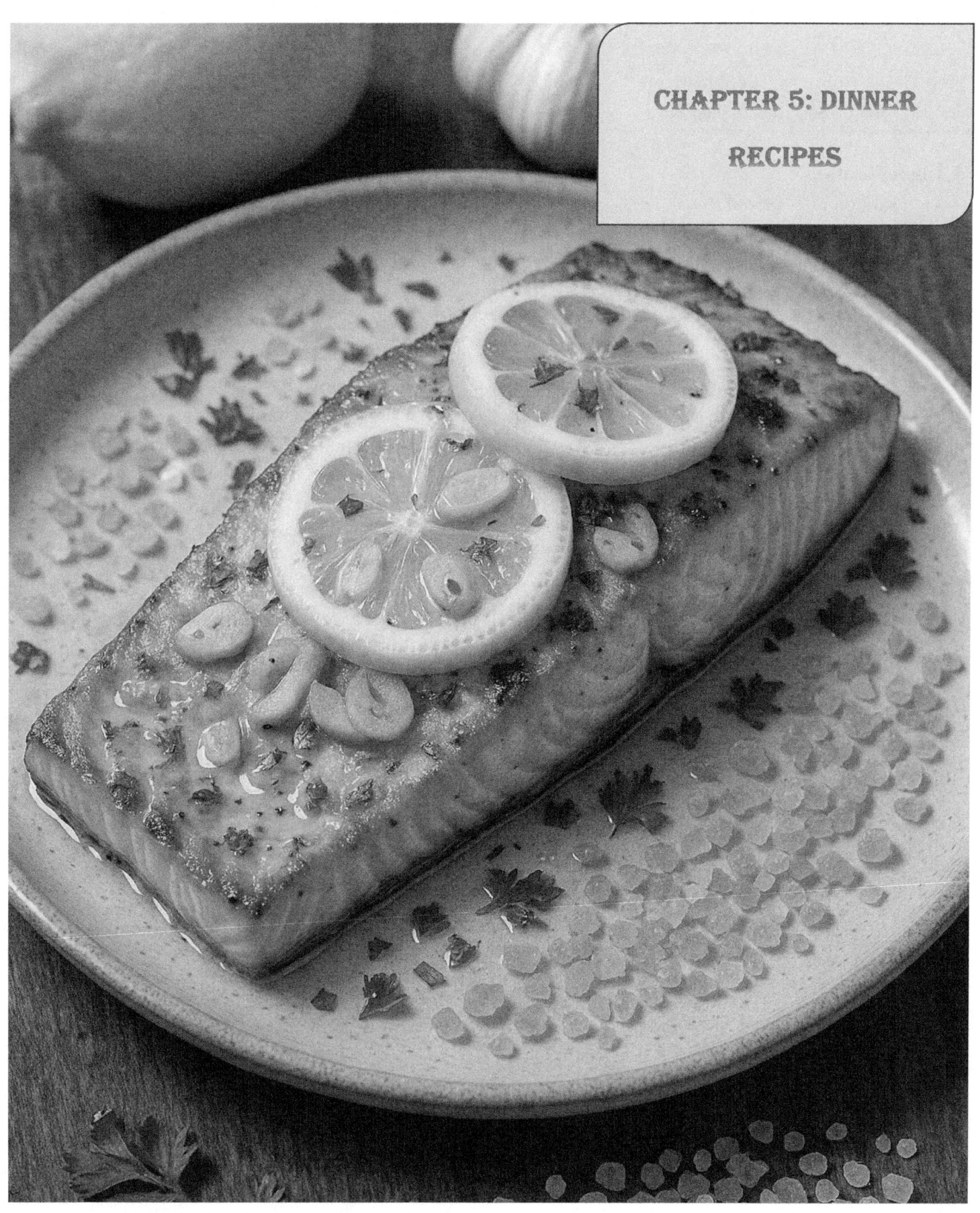

Chapter 5: Dinner Recipes

Lemon Garlic Salmon with Pink Salt

Prep Time: 5 mins | Cooking Time: 15 mins | Servings: 1 fillet

Ingredients:
- 1 salmon fillet (about 5–6 oz)
- 1 tablespoon olive oil
- 1 clove garlic, minced
- 1 tablespoon fresh lemon juice
- ½ teaspoon lemon zest
- ¼ teaspoon Himalayan pink salt
- ⅛ teaspoon black pepper
- Optional: chopped parsley for garnish
- Lemon wedges for serving

Instructions:
1. Preheat oven to 400°F (200°C). Line a baking sheet with parchment paper or foil.
2. In a small bowl, mix olive oil, garlic, lemon juice, lemon zest, pink salt, and pepper.
3. Place salmon fillet on the baking sheet and brush generously with the lemon-garlic mixture.
4. Bake for 12–15 minutes, or until salmon flakes easily with a fork.
5. Garnish with parsley and serve with lemon wedges.

Nutritional Information (per serving):

Calories: 330 | Sodium: 290 mg | Sugar: 0g | Fat: 22g | Carbs: 1g | Protein: 29g

Pink Salt Chicken Stir-Fry with Veggies

Prep Time: 10 mins | Cooking Time: 15 mins | Servings: 1 plate

Ingredients:
- 1 small chicken breast, thinly sliced
- 1 tablespoon olive oil or sesame oil
- ½ cup broccoli florets
- ¼ cup sliced bell peppers
- ¼ cup carrot matchsticks
- 1 teaspoon low-sodium soy sauce or tamari
- ¼ teaspoon Himalayan pink salt
- 1 clove garlic, minced
- ½ teaspoon grated fresh ginger
- Pinch of red pepper flakes (optional)
- 1 teaspoon fresh lemon or lime juice
- Optional: sesame seeds or green onions for garnish

Instructions:
1. Heat oil in a wok or skillet over medium-high heat. Add garlic and ginger; sauté for 30 seconds.
2. Add chicken slices and stir-fry for 4–5 minutes until cooked through and lightly browned.
3. Toss in broccoli, bell peppers, and carrots. Stir-fry for another 4–5 minutes until veggies are crisp-tender.
4. Add soy sauce, pink salt, lemon juice, and red pepper flakes if using. Stir to combine well.
5. Remove from heat and garnish with sesame seeds or green onions if desired. Serve hot.

Nutritional Information (per serving):

Calories: 320 | Sodium: 330 mg | Sugar: 5g | Fat: 16g | Carbs: 12g | Protein: 30g

Vegan Cauliflower & Chickpea Curry

Prep Time: 10 mins | Cooking Time: 20 mins | Servings: 1 bowl

Ingredients:
- ½ cup canned chickpeas, rinsed and drained
- 1 cup cauliflower florets
- ½ small onion, chopped
- 1 clove garlic, minced
- ½ teaspoon grated fresh ginger
- ½ teaspoon ground turmeric
- ½ teaspoon curry powder
- ¼ teaspoon Himalayan pink salt
- ⅛ teaspoon black pepper
- ½ cup canned coconut milk
- ¼ cup diced tomatoes
- 1 teaspoon olive oil
- Optional: fresh cilantro for garnish
- Optional: cooked brown rice or quinoa for serving

Instructions:
1. Heat olive oil in a pan over medium heat. Sauté onion for 3–4 minutes until translucent.
2. Add garlic and ginger; cook for 1 minute until fragrant.
3. Stir in turmeric, curry powder, pink salt, and pepper. Mix well.
4. Add cauliflower florets and chickpeas. Stir to coat with the spices.
5. Pour in coconut milk and diced tomatoes. Bring to a gentle simmer.
6. Cover and cook for 15–20 minutes, or until cauliflower is tender.
7. Serve warm, topped with fresh cilantro and optionally over brown rice or quinoa.

Nutritional Information (per serving, without rice):
Calories: 310 | Sodium: 320 mg | Sugar: 5g | Fat: 18g | Carbs: 26g | Protein: 8g

Baked Pink Salted Cod with Citrus Zest

Prep Time: 10 mins | Cooking Time: 15 mins | Servings: 1 fillet

Ingredients:
- 1 cod fillet (5–6 oz)
- 1 tablespoon olive oil
- 1 teaspoon lemon zest
- ½ teaspoon orange zest
- 1 tablespoon fresh lemon juice
- 1 clove garlic, minced
- ¼ teaspoon Himalayan pink salt
- ⅛ teaspoon black pepper
- Optional: chopped parsley for garnish
- Lemon or orange wedges for serving

Instructions:
1. Preheat oven to 400°F (200°C) and line a baking dish with parchment paper.
2. In a small bowl, whisk together olive oil, lemon zest, orange zest, lemon juice, garlic, pink salt, and pepper.
3. Place the cod fillet in the baking dish and spoon the citrus mixture over the top.
4. Bake for 12–15 minutes, or until the fish flakes easily with a fork.
5. Garnish with chopped parsley and serve with citrus wedges on the side.

Nutritional Information (per serving):
Calories: 270 | Sodium: 280 mg | Sugar: 1g | Fat: 15g | Carbs: 2g | Protein: 29g

Roasted Turkey Meatballs with Pink Salt

Prep Time: 10 mins ⏲ | Cooking Time: 20 mins 🔥 | Servings: 2 portions (6 meatballs) 🍽

📝 Ingredients:
- ½ lb (225g) lean ground turkey 🦃
- 1 tablespoon finely chopped onion 🧅
- 1 clove garlic, minced 🧄
- 1 tablespoon chopped parsley 🌿
- 1 tablespoon oat flour or almond flour 🌾
- 1 tablespoon grated Parmesan cheese (optional) 🧀
- 1 teaspoon olive oil 🫒
- ¼ teaspoon Himalayan pink salt 🧂
- ⅛ teaspoon black pepper 🌶
- ¼ teaspoon dried oregano or Italian seasoning 🌿

👨‍🍳 Instructions:
1. Preheat oven to 400°F (200°C). Line a baking sheet with parchment paper.
2. In a bowl, mix all ingredients until well combined.
3. Roll mixture into 1-inch balls (about 6 total) and place on the baking sheet.
4. Lightly brush or spray with olive oil.
5. Roast for 18–20 minutes, turning once halfway through, until golden and cooked through.
6. Serve warm with your favorite pink salt side or dipping sauce.

🔍 Nutritional Information (per serving – 3 meatballs):
Calories: 220 🔥 | Sodium: 310 mg 🧂 | Sugar: 1g 🍭 | Fat: 13g 🧈 | Carbs: 3g 🍚 | Protein: 22g 🍖

Stir-Fried Tofu and Broccoli in Pink Salt Sauce

Prep Time: 10 mins ⏲ | Cooking Time: 15 mins 🔥 | Servings: 1 bowl 🍽

📝 Ingredients:
- ½ block firm tofu (about 150g), pressed and cubed 🧽
- 1 cup broccoli florets 🥦
- 1 tablespoon olive oil or sesame oil 🫒
- 1 clove garlic, minced 🧄
- ½ teaspoon grated ginger 🌱
- ¼ teaspoon Himalayan pink salt 🧂
- 1 tablespoon low-sodium soy sauce or tamari 🍶
- 1 teaspoon rice vinegar 🥣
- ½ teaspoon maple syrup or honey 🍯
- 1 teaspoon cornstarch (optional, for thicker sauce)
- 2 tablespoons water 💧
- Optional: sesame seeds or chopped scallions for garnish 🌿

👨‍🍳 Instructions:
1. In a small bowl, whisk together soy sauce, rice vinegar, maple syrup, pink salt, and water. Add cornstarch if using and stir until smooth. Set aside.
2. Heat oil in a large skillet or wok over medium-high heat. Add tofu and cook until golden on all sides, about 6–8 minutes. Remove from pan and set aside.
3. Add broccoli to the same pan and stir-fry for 3–4 minutes until tender-crisp.
4. Return tofu to the pan. Add garlic and ginger, stir-fry for 1 minute.
5. Pour in the sauce and cook for another 1–2 minutes until everything is well coated and the sauce thickens.
6. Serve warm, garnished with sesame seeds or scallions.

🔍 Nutritional Information (per serving):
Calories: 320 🔥 | Sodium: 340 mg 🧂 | Sugar: 4g 🍭 | Fat: 20g 🧈 | Carbs: 18g 🍚 | Protein: 15g 🍖

Grilled Eggplant with Pink Salt Herb Drizzle

Prep Time: 10 mins | Cooking Time: 15 mins | Servings: 2 slices

📝 Ingredients:
- 1 small eggplant, sliced into ½-inch rounds
- 1 tablespoon olive oil
- ¼ teaspoon Himalayan pink salt
- ⅛ teaspoon black pepper
- For the Herb Drizzle:
- 1 tablespoon olive oil
- 1 teaspoon fresh lemon juice
- 1 tablespoon chopped parsley
- 1 teaspoon chopped mint or basil (optional)
- ¼ teaspoon Himalayan pink salt
- 1 small garlic clove, finely grated

👨‍🍳 Instructions:
1. Preheat a grill or grill pan over medium heat.
2. Brush eggplant slices with olive oil and season with pink salt and pepper.
3. Grill for 4–5 minutes on each side, until tender and grill-marked.
4. In a small bowl, mix all herb drizzle ingredients until well combined.
5. Arrange grilled eggplant on a plate and spoon the herb drizzle over the top.
6. Serve warm or at room temperature.

🔍 Nutritional Information (per serving – 2 slices with drizzle):
Calories: 180 | Sodium: 290 mg | Sugar: 4g | Fat: 15g | Carbs: 10g | Protein: 2g

Sautéed Spinach & Mushrooms with Pink Salt

Prep Time: 5 mins | Cooking Time: 10 mins | Servings: 1 plate

📝 Ingredients:
- 1 cup fresh spinach leaves
- ½ cup sliced mushrooms (button or cremini)
- 1 tablespoon olive oil or avocado oil
- 1 clove garlic, minced
- ¼ teaspoon Himalayan pink salt
- ⅛ teaspoon black pepper
- Optional: pinch of red pepper flakes
- Optional: squeeze of lemon juice

👨‍🍳 Instructions:
1. Heat oil in a skillet over medium heat. Add garlic and sauté for 30 seconds.
2. Add mushrooms and cook for 4–5 minutes, stirring occasionally, until browned and tender.
3. Add spinach and cook for 1–2 minutes, stirring, until wilted.
4. Season with pink salt, black pepper, and optional red pepper flakes.
5. Finish with a light squeeze of lemon juice if desired. Serve warm as a side or topping.

🔍 Nutritional Information (per serving):
Calories: 140 | Sodium: 280 mg | Sugar: 2g | Fat: 11g | Carbs: 6g | Protein: 3g

Zucchini Noodles with Pink Salt Tomato Sauce

Prep Time: 10 mins ⏱ | Cooking Time: 10 mins 🔥 | Servings: 1 bowl 🍽

📝 Ingredients:

For the Zucchini Noodles:
- 1 medium zucchini, spiralized 🥒
- 1 teaspoon olive oil 🫒
- Pinch of Himalayan pink salt 🧂

For the Tomato Sauce:
- ½ cup crushed tomatoes 🍅
- 1 small garlic clove, minced 🧄
- 1 tablespoon chopped onion 🧅
- 1 teaspoon olive oil 🫒
- ¼ teaspoon Himalayan pink salt 🧂
- ¼ teaspoon dried oregano 🌿
- ⅛ teaspoon black pepper 🌶
- Optional: pinch of red pepper flakes 🌶
- Optional: fresh basil for garnish 🌿

👨‍🍳 Instructions:

1. Heat 1 tsp olive oil in a skillet. Add zucchini noodles and sauté for 1–2 minutes until just tender. Season with a pinch of pink salt. Remove and set aside.
2. In the same skillet, heat 1 tbsp olive oil. Add onion and garlic, sauté for 2–3 minutes until fragrant.
3. Add crushed tomatoes, pink salt, oregano, black pepper, and optional red pepper flakes. Simmer for 5 minutes, stirring occasionally.
4. Pour sauce over the zucchini noodles and toss gently.
5. Garnish with fresh basil if desired and serve warm.

🔍 Nutritional Information (per serving):

Calories: 140 🔥 | Sodium: 300 mg 🧂 | Sugar: 7g 🔍 | Fat: 10g 🧈 | Carbs: 10g 🍞 | Protein: 3g 🔍

Herbed Basmati Rice with Pink Salt

Prep Time: 5 mins ⏱ | Cooking Time: 15 mins 🔥 | Servings: 1 bowl 🍽

📝 Ingredients:

- ½ cup basmati rice, rinsed 🌾
- 1 cup water 💧
- ¼ teaspoon Himalayan pink salt 🧂
- 1 teaspoon olive oil or unsalted butter 🧈
- 1 tablespoon chopped fresh parsley 🌿
- 1 teaspoon chopped fresh dill or cilantro (optional) 🌿
- Optional: ½ teaspoon lemon zest 🍋

👨‍🍳 Instructions:

1. In a saucepan, bring water to a boil. Add rinsed rice, pink salt, and olive oil or butter.
2. Reduce heat to low, cover, and simmer for 12–15 minutes, or until water is absorbed and rice is tender.
3. Remove from heat and let it sit, covered, for 5 minutes.
4. Fluff rice with a fork and stir in chopped herbs and optional lemon zest.
5. Serve warm as a side dish or a base for mains.

🔍 Nutritional Information (per serving):

Calories: 210 🔥 | Sodium: 290 mg 🧂 | Sugar: 0g 🔍 | Fat: 5g 🧈 | Carbs: 38g 🍞 | Protein: 4g 🔍

Pink Salt Chili Lime Chicken Skewers

Prep Time: 10 mins | Cooking Time: 15 mins | Servings: 2 skewers

Ingredients:
- 1 small chicken breast, cut into cubes
- 1 tablespoon olive oil
- 1 tablespoon fresh lime juice
- ½ teaspoon lime zest
- ¼ teaspoon Himalayan pink salt
- ¼ teaspoon chili powder
- 1 small garlic clove, minced
- Optional: chopped cilantro for garnish
- 2 wooden or metal skewers

Instructions:
1. In a bowl, combine olive oil, lime juice, lime zest, pink salt, chili powder, and garlic.
2. Add chicken cubes and toss to coat. Marinate for at least 10 minutes (or up to 2 hours for more flavor).
3. Preheat grill or grill pan over medium-high heat.
4. Thread marinated chicken onto skewers.
5. Grill skewers for 12–15 minutes, turning occasionally, until chicken is cooked through and slightly charred.
6. Garnish with fresh cilantro and serve with lime wedges.

Nutritional Information (per serving – 1 skewer):
Calories: 190 | Sodium: 280 mg | Sugar: 0g | Fat: 10g | Carbs: 1g | Protein: 22g

Stuffed Zucchini Boats with Pink Salt

Prep Time: 10 mins | Cooking Time: 25 mins | Servings: 2 boats

Ingredients:
- 1 medium zucchini, halved lengthwise and scooped
- ¼ cup cooked quinoa or brown rice
- ¼ cup canned black beans, rinsed and drained
- ¼ cup diced tomatoes
- 1 tablespoon chopped red onion
- 1 clove garlic, minced
- ½ teaspoon cumin
- ¼ teaspoon smoked paprika
- ¼ teaspoon Himalayan pink salt
- 1 teaspoon olive oil
- Optional: shredded cheese for topping
- Optional: chopped cilantro for garnish

Instructions:
1. Preheat oven to 375°F (190°C). Line a baking dish with parchment paper.
2. Brush zucchini halves with olive oil and place in the baking dish.
3. In a bowl, combine quinoa or rice, black beans, tomatoes, onion, garlic, cumin, paprika, and pink salt. Mix well.
4. Spoon the mixture into the hollowed zucchini halves.
5. Top with shredded cheese if using.
6. Cover with foil and bake for 20–25 minutes, until zucchini is tender.
7. Garnish with chopped cilantro and serve warm.

Nutritional Information (per serving – 1 stuffed boat):
Calories: 180 | Sodium: 290 mg | Sugar: 4g | Fat: 7g | Carbs: 20g | Protein: 7g

Moroccan Chickpea Stew with Pink Salt

Prep Time: 10 mins | Cooking Time: 25 mins | Servings: 1 bowl

Ingredients:
- ½ cup canned chickpeas, rinsed and drained
- ¼ cup diced carrots
- ¼ cup chopped tomatoes
- ¼ cup chopped onion
- 1 clove garlic, minced
- ½ teaspoon ground cumin
- ¼ teaspoon ground cinnamon
- ¼ teaspoon ground turmeric
- ¼ teaspoon smoked paprika
- ¼ teaspoon Himalayan pink salt
- 1 cup vegetable broth or water
- 1 tablespoon olive oil
- Optional: chopped fresh cilantro or parsley for garnish
- Optional: lemon wedge for serving

Instructions:
1. Heat olive oil in a medium pot over medium heat. Add onions and carrots; sauté for 4–5 minutes until softened.
2. Stir in garlic, cumin, cinnamon, turmeric, paprika, and pink salt. Cook for 1 minute until fragrant.
3. Add chickpeas, tomatoes, and broth. Stir well and bring to a simmer.
4. Cover and cook for 15–20 minutes, stirring occasionally, until the stew thickens slightly and flavors meld.
5. Taste and adjust seasoning if needed. Serve warm with optional herbs and lemon.

Nutritional Information (per serving):
Calories: 260 | Sodium: 310 mg | Sugar: 6g | Fat: 10g | Carbs: 32g | Protein: 9g

Thai-Inspired Pink Salt Coconut Soup

Prep Time: 10 mins | Cooking Time: 15 mins | Servings: 1 bowl

Ingredients:
- ½ cup canned coconut milk
- ½ cup vegetable broth or water
- ¼ cup sliced mushrooms
- ¼ cup diced tofu or shredded cooked chicken (optional)
- 1 tablespoon lime juice
- 1 teaspoon grated fresh ginger
- 1 clove garlic, minced
- ¼ teaspoon Himalayan pink salt
- 1 teaspoon soy sauce or tamari
- 1 small chili or pinch of chili flakes (optional)
- 1 tablespoon chopped cilantro or Thai basil

Instructions:
1. In a medium saucepan, combine coconut milk, broth, ginger, garlic, and pink salt.
2. Bring to a gentle simmer over medium heat.
3. Add mushrooms and tofu (or chicken if using). Simmer for 7–10 minutes, until mushrooms are tender.
4. Stir in lime juice, soy sauce, and chili (if using). Simmer 1–2 more minutes.
5. Serve hot, garnished with chopped herbs.

Nutritional Information (per serving):
Calories: 220 | Sodium: 300 mg | Sugar: 3g | Fat: 18g | Carbs: 10g | Protein: 5g

Teriyaki Glazed Tempeh with Pink Salt

Prep Time: 10 mins | Cooking Time: 15 mins | Servings: 1 plate

📝 Ingredients:

For the Tempeh:
- ½ block tempeh (about 100g), sliced into thin strips
- 1 teaspoon olive oil or sesame oil
- ¼ teaspoon Himalayan pink salt

For the Teriyaki Glaze:
- 1 tablespoon low-sodium soy sauce or tamari
- 1 teaspoon maple syrup or honey
- ½ teaspoon rice vinegar
- ¼ teaspoon grated fresh ginger
- ¼ teaspoon minced garlic
- 2 tablespoons water
- ¼ teaspoon cornstarch (optional, for thickness)
- Optional for garnish:
- Sesame seeds
- Chopped green onions

👩‍🍳 Instructions:

1. Steam tempeh for 5 minutes to remove bitterness. Pat dry.
2. Heat oil in a skillet over medium heat. Add tempeh and pink salt. Pan-fry for 6–8 minutes until golden and crisp, flipping halfway.
3. In a small bowl, whisk together soy sauce, maple syrup, vinegar, ginger, garlic, water, and cornstarch.
4. Pour glaze into the pan with tempeh. Cook for 2–3 minutes, stirring, until sauce thickens and tempeh is well coated.
5. Remove from heat and garnish with sesame seeds and green onions if desired. Serve warm.

🔍 Nutritional Information (per serving):

Calories: 230 | Sodium: 300 mg | Sugar: 4g | Fat: 14g | Carbs: 12g | Protein: 15g

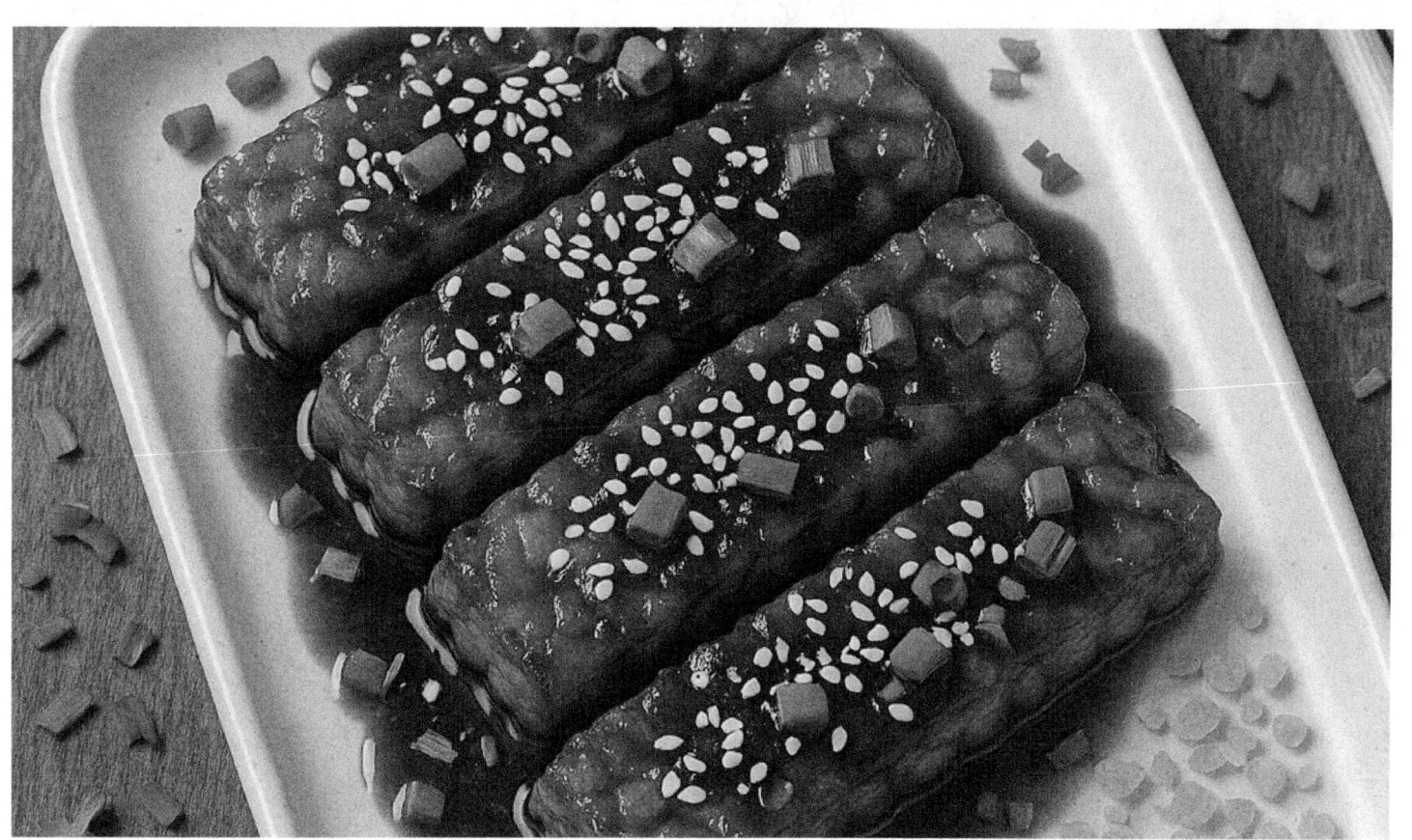

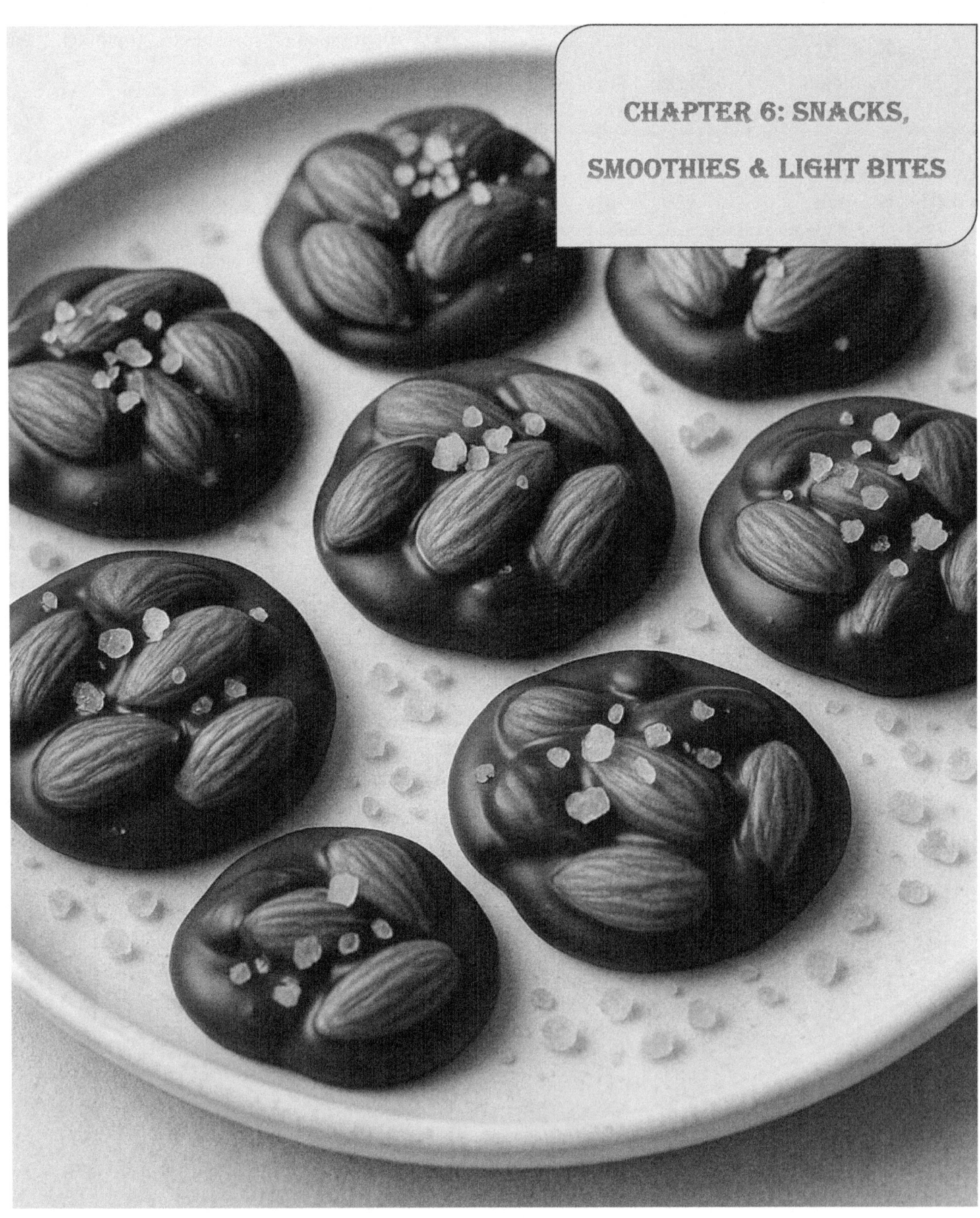

CHAPTER 6: SNACKS, SMOOTHIES & LIGHT BITES

Pink Salt Dark Chocolate Almond Bites

Prep Time: 5 mins | Cooking Time: 5 mins (plus chilling) | Servings: 6 bites

Ingredients:
- ½ cup whole raw almonds
- ¼ cup dark chocolate chips or chopped dark chocolate (70% or higher)
- ¼ teaspoon Himalayan pink salt, plus extra for topping
- ½ teaspoon coconut oil (optional, for smoother melting)

Instructions:
1. Line a plate or small tray with parchment paper.
2. Melt the dark chocolate and coconut oil (if using) in a microwave or double boiler until smooth.
3. Stir in the pink salt and almonds until almonds are fully coated.
4. Spoon small clusters onto the parchment paper.
5. Sprinkle a tiny pinch of extra pink salt over each bite.
6. Chill in the refrigerator for 20–30 minutes or until set.
7. Store in an airtight container in the fridge.

Nutritional Information (per bite):
Calories: 95 | Sodium: 85 mg | Sugar: 3g | Fat: 7g | Carbs: 6g | Protein: 2g

Pink Salt Sweet Potato Chips

Prep Time: 5 mins | Cooking Time: 20 mins | Servings: 1 bowl

Ingredients:
- 1 medium sweet potato, thinly sliced (use a mandoline for best results)
- 1 tablespoon olive oil or avocado oil
- ¼ teaspoon Himalayan pink salt
- Optional: pinch of smoked paprika or cayenne pepper

Instructions:
1. Preheat oven to 375°F (190°C) and line a baking sheet with parchment paper.
2. In a bowl, toss sweet potato slices with oil, pink salt, and optional spices.
3. Arrange slices in a single layer on the baking sheet, ensuring they don't overlap.
4. Bake for 18–22 minutes, flipping halfway through, until crispy and golden.
5. Remove and let cool slightly—they'll crisp up more as they cool.
6. Enjoy immediately or store in an airtight container for up to 2 days.

Nutritional Information (per serving):
Calories: 160 | Sodium: 280 mg | Sugar: 4g | Fat: 7g | Carbs: 22g | Protein: 2g

Avocado Salsa with Pink Salt

Prep Time: 10 mins | Cooking Time: 0 mins | Servings: 1 bowl

Ingredients:
- 1 ripe avocado, diced
- ¼ cup cherry tomatoes, diced
- 2 tablespoons red onion, finely chopped
- 1 tablespoon fresh lime juice
- 1 tablespoon fresh cilantro, chopped
- ¼ teaspoon Himalayan pink salt
- ⅛ teaspoon black pepper
- Optional: ½ jalapeño, finely chopped for heat

Instructions:
1. In a bowl, gently combine diced avocado, tomatoes, red onion, and optional jalapeño.
2. Add lime juice, pink salt, pepper, and cilantro. Toss gently to combine.
3. Serve immediately with veggie sticks, whole grain crackers, or as a topping for bowls and wraps.

Nutritional Information (per serving):
Calories: 160 | Sodium: 290 mg | Sugar: 2g | Fat: 13g | Carbs: 10g | Protein: 2g

Pink Salt Edamame Pods

Prep Time: 5 mins | Cooking Time: 5 mins | Servings: 1 bowl

Ingredients:
- 1 cup frozen edamame pods (in-shell)
- ½ teaspoon Himalayan pink salt
- Optional: a drizzle of sesame oil or a pinch of chili flakes for extra flavor

Instructions:
1. Bring a pot of water to a boil. Add edamame and cook for 4–5 minutes until tender.
2. Drain and transfer to a bowl.
3. Sprinkle with pink salt and toss to coat evenly.
4. Add sesame oil or chili flakes if using, then serve warm or at room temperature.
5. To eat: pop the beans out of the pod with your teeth and discard the shell.

Nutritional Information (per serving):
Calories: 140 | Sodium: 280 mg | Sugar: 2g | Fat: 5g | Carbs: 12g | Protein: 12g

Spiced Carrot Hummus with Pink Salt

Prep Time: 10 mins | Cooking Time: 20 mins | Servings: 1 bowl

Ingredients:
- 1 cup chopped carrots
- ½ cup canned chickpeas, rinsed and drained
- 1 tablespoon tahini
- 1 tablespoon olive oil
- 1 tablespoon lemon juice
- 1 clove garlic, minced
- ¼ teaspoon ground cumin
- ¼ teaspoon ground coriander
- ¼ teaspoon Himalayan pink salt
- 2 tablespoons water (as needed for blending)
- Optional: pinch of cayenne or paprika for extra heat

Instructions:
1. Steam or boil chopped carrots for 15–20 minutes until very tender. Let cool slightly.
2. In a food processor, combine cooked carrots, chickpeas, tahini, olive oil, lemon juice, garlic, cumin, coriander, and pink salt.
3. Blend until smooth, adding water gradually to reach desired consistency.
4. Taste and adjust seasoning as needed.
5. Transfer to a bowl, garnish with a drizzle of olive oil and optional paprika. Serve with veggie sticks or whole grain crackers.

Nutritional Information (per serving):

Calories: 180 | Sodium: 270 mg | Sugar: 5g | Fat: 9g | Carbs: 18g | Protein: 5g

---

Pink Salt Nut & Seed Trail Mix

Prep Time: 5 mins | Cooking Time: 0 mins | Servings: 1 handful (about ¼ cup)

Ingredients:
- 2 tablespoons raw almonds
- 2 tablespoons raw cashews
- 1 tablespoon pumpkin seeds (pepitas)
- 1 tablespoon sunflower seeds
- 1 tablespoon dried cranberries or raisins
- 1 teaspoon chia seeds
- ¼ teaspoon Himalayan pink salt
- Optional: pinch of cinnamon or cacao nibs for extra flavor

Instructions:
1. In a mixing bowl, combine all nuts, seeds, and dried fruit.
2. Sprinkle with Himalayan pink salt and toss well to coat evenly.
3. Add cinnamon or cacao nibs if using for added flavor.
4. Store in an airtight container or resealable snack bag for on-the-go energy!

Nutritional Information (per serving – ¼ cup):

Calories: 190 | Sodium: 200 mg | Sugar: 4g | Fat: 14g | Carbs: 12g | Protein: 5g

Detox Smoothie with Cucumber, Mint & Pink Salt

Prep Time: 5 mins ⏱ | Cooking Time: 0 mins ❄ | Servings: 1 glass 🥤

📝 Ingredients:
- ½ cucumber, peeled and chopped
- 5–6 fresh mint leaves
- ½ green apple, chopped
- Juice of ½ lemon
- ¾ cup cold water or unsweetened coconut water
- ¼ teaspoon Himalayan pink salt
- A few ice cubes

👨‍🍳 Instructions:
1. Add all ingredients to a blender.
2. Blend on high until smooth and frothy.
3. Taste and adjust lemon or salt if needed.
4. Serve immediately for a refreshing detox boost!

🔍 Nutritional Information (per serving):
Calories: 60 | Sodium: 290 mg | Sugar: 7g | Fat: 0g | Carbs: 13g | Protein: 1g

Pink Salt Watermelon & Mint Salad

Prep Time: 5 mins ⏱ | Cooking Time: 0 mins ❄ | Servings: 1 bowl 🍽

📝 Ingredients:
- 1 cup watermelon, cubed
- 1 tablespoon fresh mint leaves, chopped
- ¼ teaspoon Himalayan pink salt
- ½ teaspoon fresh lime juice
- Optional: pinch of chili flakes for a spicy kick
- Optional: sprinkle of crumbled feta cheese

👨‍🍳 Instructions:
1. In a bowl, combine cubed watermelon and chopped mint.
2. Drizzle with lime juice and sprinkle with Himalayan pink salt.
3. Add chili flakes or feta if desired, and toss gently.
4. Serve immediately while chilled and juicy.

🔍 Nutritional Information (per serving):
Calories: 50 | Sodium: 290 mg | Sugar: 9g | Fat: 0g | Carbs: 11g | Protein: 1g

Protein Bars with Pink Salt & Cranberries

Prep Time: 10 mins | Cooking Time: 0 mins (chill for 30 mins) | Servings: 4 bars

Ingredients:
- ½ cup rolled oats
- ¼ cup protein powder (vanilla or unflavored)
- 2 tablespoons almond butter or peanut butter
- 2 tablespoons honey or maple syrup
- 2 tablespoons dried cranberries
- 1 tablespoon chia seeds
- ¼ teaspoon Himalayan pink salt
- 1 tablespoon water or almond milk (if needed)

Instructions:
1. In a mixing bowl, combine oats, protein powder, cranberries, chia seeds, and pink salt.
2. In a separate bowl, warm the nut butter and honey/maple syrup until easily mixable.
3. Pour the wet mixture into the dry ingredients and stir until combined. Add a splash of water or almond milk if too dry.
4. Press the mixture firmly into a small lined container or dish.
5. Chill in the fridge for 30 minutes, then cut into bars.
6. Store in an airtight container in the fridge for up to 5 days.

Nutritional Information (per bar):
Calories: 180 | Sodium: 140 mg | Sugar: 7g | Fat: 8g | Carbs: 18g | Protein: 9g

Spicy Pink Salt Roasted Chickpeas

Prep Time: 5 mins | Cooking Time: 30 mins | Servings: 1 cup

Ingredients:
- 1 cup canned chickpeas, rinsed, drained, and patted dry
- 1 tablespoon olive oil
- ¼ teaspoon Himalayan pink salt
- ½ teaspoon smoked paprika
- ¼ teaspoon cayenne pepper or chili powder
- ¼ teaspoon garlic powder
- Optional: pinch of black pepper

Instructions:
1. Preheat oven to 400°F (200°C) and line a baking sheet with parchment paper.
2. In a bowl, toss the chickpeas with olive oil, pink salt, paprika, cayenne, garlic powder, and black pepper (if using).
3. Spread chickpeas out in a single layer on the baking sheet.
4. Roast for 25–30 minutes, shaking the pan halfway through, until crispy and golden.
5. Let cool slightly before enjoying as a crunchy, high-protein snack.

Nutritional Information (per serving – 1 cup):
Calories: 210 | Sodium: 300 mg | Sugar: 2g | Fat: 10g | Carbs: 24g | Protein: 9g

Strawberry Coconut Shake with Pink Salt

Prep Time: 5 mins | Cooking Time: 0 mins | Servings: 1 glass

Ingredients:
- 1 cup frozen strawberries
- ½ cup coconut milk (unsweetened)
- ¼ cup water
- 1 tablespoon honey or maple syrup
- ¼ teaspoon Himalayan pink salt
- ½ teaspoon vanilla extract
- Optional: 1 tablespoon chia seeds or ground flaxseeds
- Ice cubes (optional for extra thickness)

Instructions:
1. Combine all ingredients (strawberries, coconut milk, water, honey, pink salt, and vanilla) in a blender.
2. Blend on high until smooth and creamy.
3. Add ice cubes if you prefer a thicker texture, and blend again.
4. Serve immediately for a refreshing, hydrating treat.

Nutritional Information (per serving):
Calories: 180 | Sodium: 290 mg | Sugar: 15g | Fat: 10g | Carbs: 20g | Protein: 2g

Almond-Coconut Balls with a Pink Salt Twist

Prep Time: 10 mins | Cooking Time: 0 mins | Servings: 6 balls

Ingredients:
- 1 cup unsweetened shredded coconut
- ½ cup almonds, finely chopped or ground
- 2 tablespoons almond butter or peanut butter
- 1 tablespoon honey or maple syrup
- ¼ teaspoon Himalayan pink salt
- 1 teaspoon vanilla extract
- Optional: 1 tablespoon chia seeds or flaxseeds

Instructions:
1. In a bowl, combine shredded coconut, chopped almonds, almond butter, honey, pink salt, and vanilla extract.
2. Stir everything together until well combined.
3. Roll the mixture into small balls (about 1 tablespoon each).
4. Chill in the refrigerator for 20–30 minutes to set.
5. Serve and enjoy as a quick, energy-boosting snack!

Nutritional Information (per serving – 1 ball):
Calories: 160 | Sodium: 150 mg | Sugar: 5g | Fat: 12g | Carbs: 12g | Protein: 4g

Green Smoothie with Lemon & Pink Salt

Prep Time: 5 mins | Cooking Time: 0 mins | Servings: 1 glass

📝 Ingredients:
- 1 cup spinach or kale (fresh or frozen)
- ½ frozen banana
- ½ cup unsweetened almond milk (or milk of choice)
- 1 tablespoon fresh lemon juice
- ¼ teaspoon Himalayan pink salt
- ½ teaspoon chia seeds or flaxseeds (optional)
- 1 teaspoon honey or maple syrup (optional)
- Ice cubes (optional, for extra chill)

👨‍🍳 Instructions:
1. Add spinach, banana, almond milk, lemon juice, pink salt, and chia or flaxseeds (if using) to a blender.
2. Blend on high until smooth and creamy.
3. Add honey or maple syrup for sweetness, if desired, and blend again.
4. Pour into a glass and serve immediately for a refreshing, energizing drink.

🔍 Nutritional Information (per serving):
Calories: 120 | Sodium: 290 mg | Sugar: 12g | Fat: 4g | Carbs: 20g | Protein: 3g

Roasted Seaweed Snack with Pink Salt

Prep Time: 5 mins | Cooking Time: 5 mins | Servings: 1 snack pack

📝 Ingredients:
- 1 sheet roasted seaweed (nori)
- ½ teaspoon olive oil
- ¼ teaspoon Himalayan pink salt
- ¼ teaspoon sesame seeds (optional)

👨‍🍳 Instructions:
1. Preheat your oven to 350°F (175°C).
2. Lightly brush one side of the seaweed sheet with olive oil.
3. Sprinkle with pink salt and sesame seeds (if using).
4. Place the seaweed sheet on a baking sheet and bake for 3–5 minutes, until crisp.
5. Remove from the oven and let cool before breaking into pieces.
6. Serve as a healthy, savory snack!

🔍 Nutritional Information (per serving – 1 sheet):
Calories: 30 | Sodium: 200 mg | Sugar: 0g | Fat: 2g | Carbs: 2g | Protein: 1g

Frozen Banana Bites with Pink Salt & Cocoa

Prep Time: 10 mins | Cooking Time: 0 mins | Servings: 6 bites

Ingredients:
- 1 large ripe banana, sliced into ½-inch rounds
- 2 tablespoons dark chocolate chips or cocoa nibs
- 1 tablespoon almond butter or peanut butter
- ¼ teaspoon Himalayan pink salt
- 1 teaspoon cocoa powder
- Optional: 1 tablespoon shredded coconut

Instructions:
1. Lay the banana slices on a parchment-lined tray.
2. Melt the almond butter or peanut butter slightly in the microwave for 20-30 seconds until spreadable.
3. Spread a small amount of the melted nut butter onto each banana slice.
4. Sprinkle with a pinch of pink salt, cocoa powder, and optional coconut or cocoa nibs.
5. Freeze for 2–3 hours or until firm.
6. Serve immediately as a refreshing snack or store in an airtight container in the freezer for later.

Nutritional Information (per serving – 1 bite):
Calories: 60 | Sodium: 90 mg | Sugar: 5g | Fat: 3g | Carbs: 9g | Protein: 1g

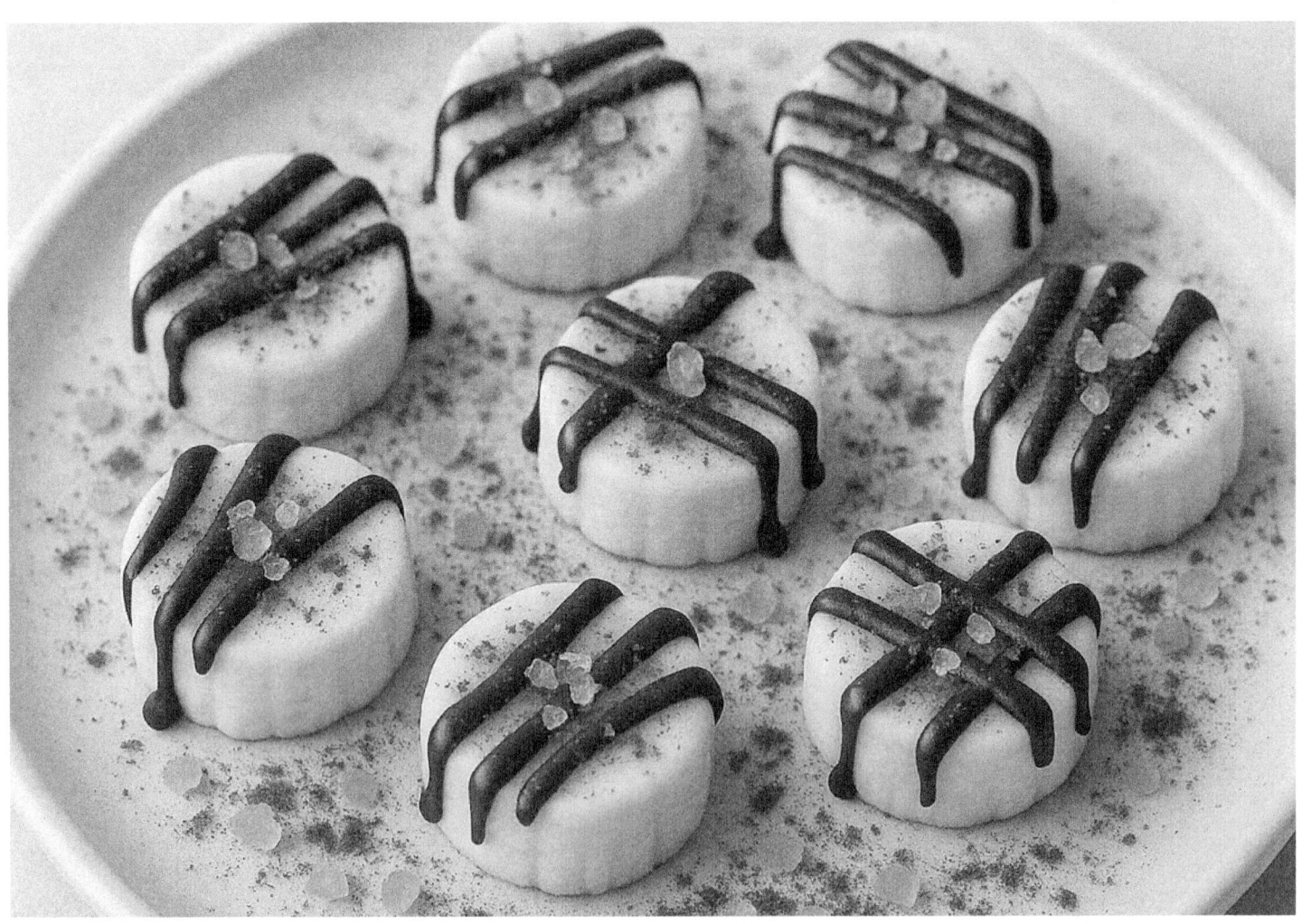

CHAPTER 7: THE 30-DAY PINK SALT TRICK MEAL PLAN

How to Follow the 30-Day Plan

Embarking on the Pink Salt Trick Diet is about more than just adding a pinch of Himalayan pink salt to your meals. It's a journey that encompasses mindful eating, balanced hydration, and a holistic approach to wellness. This 30-day plan is designed to make this transition smooth, enjoyable, and sustainable. Here's how to follow the plan for optimal results.

1. Understand the Basics

The Pink Salt Trick Diet is based on the power of Himalayan pink salt to help with weight loss, detoxification, and metabolism boosting. Throughout the 30 days, you'll consume foods that are nutrient-dense, hydrating, and designed to support your body's natural detox processes. The key principle is to balance your electrolytes, reduce cravings, and boost your metabolism through natural, wholesome meals.

2. Start Each Day with a Pink Salt Morning Flush

Every morning, begin your day with a Pink Salt Morning Detox Water. This helps hydrate your body, balance electrolytes, and jumpstart your metabolism.

Mix ¼ to ½ teaspoon of Himalayan pink salt in 8 oz of warm water and drink it on an empty stomach.

Add fresh lemon juice if desired for extra detox benefits.

3. Meal Planning for Success

Plan Ahead: Use the 30-Day Meal Plan included in this book to set yourself up for success. Batch cook, prep your ingredients, and ensure your meals are quick and easy to prepare.

Customize: Feel free to substitute ingredients in the recipes based on what you have available or your preferences, but always try to keep the essence of the recipes intact (e.g., using lean proteins, fresh vegetables, and healthy fats).

4. Stay Hydrated

Proper hydration is critical to this diet's success. Apart from the Pink Salt Morning Flush, make sure to drink plenty of water throughout the day.

Aim for at least 8 cups of water daily, and increase your intake if you're exercising or in hot climates.

You can also enjoy herbal teas, infused waters, and natural detox drinks that are part of the meal plan.

5. Incorporate Mindful Eating

Eat Slowly: Take time to chew and savor your food. Mindful eating helps with digestion, satisfaction, and prevents overeating.

Balance Your Plate: Each meal should include a healthy balance of protein, healthy fats, and fiber to keep you feeling full and energized.

Avoid Overeating: Follow your body's hunger cues. If you're full, stop eating. The focus is on nourishing your body, not overeating.

6. Exercise and Movement

While the Pink Salt Trick Diet is designed to work well even without intense physical activity, adding in light exercise like walking, yoga, or strength training can accelerate results.

Aim for 20-30 minutes of movement a few times a week to boost circulation, help with digestion, and keep your energy levels up.

Remember, the goal is sustainable changes, not overexertion.

7. Track Your Progress

Keep a journal to track what you eat, how you feel, and any changes you notice. This will help you stay motivated and aware of how different foods and habits are impacting your body.

Pay attention to your energy levels, digestion, and cravings, and make adjustments if necessary.

8. End Your Day with a Detox Tea or Light Snack

Before bed, enjoy a calming herbal tea or a light snack to aid digestion and promote a restful sleep. Options like chamomile tea, peppermint tea, or a small handful of nuts and seeds can be soothing and help curb any late-night cravings.

9. Stick to the Plan for 30 Days

Consistency is key. Stick to the plan for the full 30 days to give your body time to adjust, detoxify, and see the results of the Pink Salt Trick.

After 30 days, you can choose to continue with the plan, adjust it for maintenance, or modify based on your personal goals.

10. Enjoy the Process

The Pink Salt Trick Diet is not just about following a strict regimen, but about creating a balanced, enjoyable lifestyle. Don't be too hard on yourself. Celebrate your small victories, enjoy the delicious meals, and embrace the positive changes that come from nourishing your body.

Calorie Guidance for Weight Loss

Understanding your calorie needs is crucial when it comes to effective and sustainable weight loss. While the Pink Salt Trick Diet focuses on nourishing your body with wholesome, whole foods, caloric intake is still an important factor. This section will help you understand how to manage your calorie intake while still enjoying the foods that support your weight loss goals.

1. Understanding Your Caloric Needs

To lose weight, you must create a caloric deficit, meaning you consume fewer calories than your body burns. However, it's important to do this in a healthy, balanced way to ensure you're still getting enough nutrients and energy for daily activities.

The general approach for weight loss is to aim for a 500-calorie deficit per day, which usually leads to a loss of about 1 pound (0.45 kg) per week. However, this varies depending on individual factors like age, gender, metabolism, and activity level.

How to Estimate Your Daily Caloric Needs:

a. Calculate Your Basal Metabolic Rate (BMR): This is the number of calories your body needs at rest to maintain basic functions like breathing, digestion, and circulation.

Use this formula for women:

$$BMR = 655 + (9.6 \times \text{weight in kg}) + (1.8 \times \text{height in cm}) - (4.7 \times \text{age})$$

And for men:

$$BMR = 66 + (13.7 \times \text{weight in kg}) + (5 \times \text{height in cm}) - (6.8 \times \text{age})$$

b. Determine Your Total Daily Energy Expenditure (TDEE): This takes into account your activity level. Multiply your BMR by an activity factor:

- Sedentary (little or no exercise): BMR × 1.2
- Lightly active (light exercise or sports 1-3 days/week): BMR × 1.375
- Moderately active (moderate exercise or sports 3-5 days/week): BMR × 1.55
- Very active (hard exercise or sports 6-7 days/week): BMR × 1.725
- Extremely active (very intense exercise, physical job, or training twice a day): BMR × 1.9

c. Create a Caloric Deficit:

Once you know your TDEE, subtract 500 calories for a safe and sustainable weight loss goal of around 1 pound per week.

2. Portion Control and Mindful Eating

While calorie counting is helpful, focusing on portion control and mindful eating is equally important. Eating the right portions will help you naturally consume fewer calories without feeling deprived.

- Use smaller plates to help manage portion sizes.
- Listen to your hunger cues: Eat when you're hungry and stop when you're satisfied.
- Avoid distractions while eating (like watching TV) to help you be more aware of your food.

3. Balancing Macronutrients for Weight Loss

In addition to managing calories, focusing on the right balance of macronutrients (protein, fats, and carbohydrates) will ensure you're getting the most from every meal.

Protein:

Protein helps to maintain muscle mass while losing fat and keeps you feeling full longer. Aim for at least 20-30% of your total daily calories from protein sources like lean meats, tofu, legumes, and dairy.

Healthy Fats:

Healthy fats are crucial for hormone balance, brain function, and overall health. Aim for about 25-35% of your daily calories from healthy fat sources like avocados, nuts, seeds, and olive oil.

Carbohydrates:

Carbs are your body's main energy source. Choose complex carbs like whole grains, fruits, and vegetables for sustained energy and fiber. Carbohydrates should make up about 40-50% of your daily calories.

4. Tracking Your Progress

Tracking your meals, snacks, and portion sizes can help you stay on top of your calorie intake and make adjustments when necessary. You can use an app like MyFitnessPal, or simply keep a food diary.

Here are a few simple guidelines to help you stay on track:

- Measure your food when possible.
- Focus on nutrient-dense foods (like the ones featured in the Pink Salt Trick Diet), rather than empty-calorie processed foods.
- Don't stress over occasional indulgences—it's about consistency, not perfection.

5. Making Adjustments Along the Way

As you progress through your 30-day plan, it's important to regularly assess how your body is responding. If you're feeling too hungry or fatigued, you may need to increase your caloric intake slightly. If you're not seeing the results you'd like, you may need to tighten your portion sizes or adjust your calorie intake.

Remember, weight loss is a gradual process, and your body needs time to adjust to the changes you're making. Consistency, along with the right amount of calories and nutrients, will get you the best results.

6. Avoiding Calorie Counting Burnout

If you find that calorie counting becomes too overwhelming or frustrating, don't worry! The goal is to build healthy habits, not make food feel like a chore. Here are a few tips to help:

- Focus on whole, unprocessed foods that naturally fit into the plan.
- Listen to your body and honor your hunger cues.
- Use portion control and mindful eating techniques.

In Summary:

- Understand your caloric needs using BMR and TDEE.
- Create a moderate caloric deficit of about 500 calories for weight loss.
- Balance your macronutrients to ensure adequate protein, healthy fats, and complex carbs.
- Track your progress and adjust as needed, but avoid burnout by practicing mindful eating and portion control.

Customization Tips (Vegetarian, Vegan, Gluten-Free)

The Pink Salt Trick Diet is designed to be flexible, so you can customize the plan to suit your dietary needs, whether you're vegetarian, vegan, gluten-free, or following any other specific dietary pattern. Here are some simple adjustments you can make while still enjoying the health benefits of this diet.

1. Vegetarian Customization

If you follow a vegetarian diet, this plan is already a great fit for you. However, there are a few key substitutions to make sure you're getting enough protein and variety:

Protein Sources:

- **Legumes & Beans:** Chickpeas, lentils, black beans, and kidney beans are great sources of protein. Use them in salads, soups, and stews.
- **Tofu & Tempeh:** These soy-based products are excellent meat alternatives. Try them in stir-fries, curries, or salads.

- **Dairy:** If you include dairy in your diet, opt for Greek yogurt, cottage cheese, and cheese as protein-rich options.
- **Eggs:** Include eggs for additional protein, especially in dishes like scrambled eggs, omelets, or frittatas.

Iron-Rich Foods:

As a vegetarian, make sure you're getting enough iron, which is abundant in foods like spinach, lentils, tofu, and fortified cereals. Pairing iron-rich foods with vitamin C (like citrus fruits) can enhance absorption.

Meal Ideas:

- Vegetarian Quinoa Salad with roasted vegetables and tahini dressing.
- Vegetarian Lentil Soup with pink salt and spices.
- Tofu Scramble with vegetables and avocado.

2. Vegan Customization

For those following a vegan diet, the Pink Salt Trick Diet can easily be adapted to eliminate all animal products while still providing optimal nutrition. Here are a few substitutions for vegan-friendly meals:

Protein Sources:

- **Legumes & Beans:** Chickpeas, black beans, lentils, and kidney beans are great plant-based protein sources.
- **Tofu & Tempeh:** These soy products are rich in protein and can be used as a meat replacement in stir-fries, salads, and curries.
- **Seitan:** Made from gluten, seitan is a highly versatile and protein-packed alternative to meat, perfect for stir-fries, wraps, and stews.
- **Nuts & Seeds:** Almonds, sunflower seeds, pumpkin seeds, and chia seeds provide healthy fats and protein.
- **Nutritional Yeast:** This is a great source of B-vitamins and a wonderful cheese alternative in vegan recipes.

Calcium & Vitamin D:

Make sure you are getting enough calcium and vitamin D, which are often found in fortified plant-based milks (almond, soy, or oat milk) and leafy greens like kale and collard greens.

Meal Ideas:

- Vegan Buddha Bowl with roasted veggies, quinoa, chickpeas, and tahini dressing.
- Lentil and Vegetable Curry with coconut milk, served with brown rice.
- Tempeh Stir-Fry with vegetables and a pink salt soy sauce glaze.

3. Gluten-Free Customization

If you follow a gluten-free diet, there are a few simple modifications to ensure that all meals are free from gluten:

Gluten-Free Grains:

- **Quinoa:** A complete protein and naturally gluten-free. Use it in salads, soups, and as a side dish.
- **Brown Rice:** Another great gluten-free grain that can be used as a base for stir-fries, bowls, and casseroles.
- **Buckwheat:** A gluten-free pseudocereal that works well in pancakes, waffles, and grain bowls.

- **Amaranth & Millet:** These gluten-free grains are perfect for soups, salads, or as a base for a hearty dish.

Gluten-Free Flours:

If you're baking or preparing dishes that require flour, opt for almond flour, coconut flour, rice flour, or gluten-free all-purpose flour.

Avoid Processed Gluten-Free Foods:

While there are many gluten-free packaged products available, they can often be highly processed and low in nutrients. Focus on whole, unprocessed foods like vegetables, fruits, legumes, nuts, and seeds.

Meal Ideas:

- Gluten-Free Tofu Scramble with quinoa and sautéed vegetables.
- Chickpea Salad with avocado, cucumber, and a lemon-pink salt dressing.
- Gluten-Free Vegetable Stir-Fry with brown rice and a tamari-pink salt glaze.

4. Combination of Dietary Preferences

If you're following a combination of dietary preferences, such as vegan and gluten-free, vegetarian and gluten-free, or other variations, here are some quick tips for easy modifications:

- **Vegetarian + Gluten-Free:** Stick with quinoa, rice, potatoes, and gluten-free grains. Add beans, lentils, and tofu for protein.
- **Vegan + Gluten-Free:** Opt for legume-based pastas, quinoa, and rice as your base. Tempeh, tofu, and chickpeas are perfect protein sources.
- **Vegan + Gluten-Free + Low-Carb:** Focus on non-starchy vegetables like cauliflower, zucchini, and leafy greens. Use seeds and nuts for protein and healthy fats.

5. General Tips for All Customizations

- **Plan Ahead:** Meal prep is key for all dietary preferences. Take time to prep grains, beans, and roasted vegetables in advance for quick meals.
- **Read Labels:** If you're buying packaged items (especially gluten-free or vegan), always check for added sugars or preservatives.
- **Flavor Boosters:** Use natural flavorings like fresh herbs, garlic, lemon, lime, and spices to enhance your meals without relying on gluten-containing or animal-based products.

6. Maintaining Balance

Whatever your dietary preference, remember that the Pink Salt Trick Diet is about balance—adequate protein, healthy fats, and nutrient-dense carbohydrates. Aim for a rainbow of vegetables and whole grains in every meal, and make sure your meals are high in fiber to keep you full and satisfied.

Weekly Shopping Lists

Week 1:

This week focuses on healthy fats, lean proteins, and fiber-rich vegetables. You'll be making smoothies, salads, and quick meals packed with nutrients to jumpstart your detox and weight loss journey.

Fresh Produce:

- 4 ripe avocados

- 2 zucchinis
- 1 large cucumber
- 3 medium sweet potatoes
- 1 head of broccoli
- 1 bunch spinach (or kale)
- 1 bunch fresh parsley
- 1 bunch fresh cilantro
- 2 lemons
- 3 tomatoes
- 1 small red onion
- 2 cloves garlic
- 1-inch piece fresh ginger
- 1 small bag of carrots
- 1 small bag of celery stalks
- 1 bunch mint
- 1 bunch green onions
- 2 limes
- 1 bag of fresh baby greens (arugula, spinach, etc.)

Frozen Produce:

- 1 bag frozen strawberries
- 1 bag frozen spinach (optional for smoothies)

Canned & Dry Goods:

- 1 can chickpeas (15 oz)
- 1 can black beans (15 oz)
- 1 can coconut milk (unsweetened)
- 1 small can of diced tomatoes (14 oz)
- 1 bag quinoa
- 1 bag brown rice
- 1 small bottle of tamari or soy sauce
- 1 bottle of olive oil
- 1 bottle of apple cider vinegar

Nuts, Seeds & Legumes:

- 1 bag chia seeds
- 1 bag almond butter
- 1 small bag sunflower seeds
- 1 small bag almonds
- 1 small bag pumpkin seeds
- 1 small bag sesame seeds

Dairy (or Dairy Alternatives):

- 1 small container of Greek yogurt (optional)
- 1 container almond milk (unsweetened)

Spices & Seasonings:

- Himalayan pink salt
- Ground black pepper
- Smoked paprika
- Ground cumin
- Ground turmeric
- Ground cinnamon
- Chili flakes (optional)
- Garlic powder
- Fresh or dried oregano

Week 2:

This week will incorporate more legumes, high-protein foods, and fiber-packed vegetables. The goal is to enhance detoxification and stabilize blood sugar.

Fresh Produce:

- 3 medium avocados
- 1 bunch kale
- 2 medium eggplants
- 1 bunch bok choy
- 3 bell peppers (red, yellow, green)
- 1 bunch asparagus
- 1 bunch fresh basil
- 3 apples
- 2 cups mushrooms
- 1 bunch fresh dill
- 1 small bag spinach
- 1 bunch carrots
- 2 cucumbers
- 1 bag sweet potatoes
- 1 bunch mint

Frozen Produce:

- 1 bag frozen peas
- 1 bag frozen mixed berries
- Canned & Dry Goods:
- 1 can chickpeas
- 1 can diced tomatoes
- 1 small can coconut milk
- 1 bag red lentils
- 1 bag brown rice
- 1 bag quinoa
- 1 bottle balsamic vinegar
- 1 bottle sesame oil

Nuts, Seeds & Legumes:

- 1 small bag hemp seeds
- 1 small bag almond butter
- 1 small bag walnuts
- 1 small bag chia seeds
- 1 bag raw cashews

Dairy (or Dairy Alternatives):

- 1 container coconut yogurt (optional)
- 1 container unsweetened almond milk

Spices & Seasonings:

- Ground coriander
- Ground cumin
- Ground cinnamon
- Himalayan pink salt
- Ground turmeric
- Ground black pepper
- Chili powder

Week 3:

In Week 3, we focus on balancing blood sugar and providing the body with sustained energy through complex carbs, healthy fats, and lean proteins.

Fresh Produce:

- 1 bunch fresh parsley
- 2 ripe avocados
- 1 bunch kale
- 2 bunches broccoli
- 2 zucchinis
- 2 tomatoes
- 1 medium cauliflower

- 1 head of garlic
- 1 small bunch fresh thyme
- 1 bag carrots
- 1 small bag spinach
- 1 bunch green onions
- 1 bag fresh cilantro
- 1 red onion
- 3 lemons

Frozen Produce:

- 1 bag frozen peas
- 1 bag frozen spinach

Canned & Dry Goods:

- 1 can black beans
- 1 can chickpeas
- 1 can coconut milk
- 1 bag quinoa
- 1 bag lentils
- 1 bottle apple cider vinegar
- 1 bottle olive oil

Nuts, Seeds & Legumes:

- 1 small bag chia seeds
- 1 bag almonds
- 1 bag sunflower seeds
- 1 small bag cashews

Dairy (or Dairy Alternatives):

- 1 container almond milk
- 1 small container coconut yogurt

Spices & Seasonings:

- Ground turmeric
- Ground coriander
- Ground cinnamon
- Ground cumin
- Himalayan pink salt
- Black pepper

Week 4:

The final week emphasizes whole grains, plant-based proteins, and hydration to support your body's ongoing detoxification process and enhance the benefits of the diet.

Fresh Produce:

- 1 bunch kale
- 2 ripe avocados
- 1 bunch asparagus
- 1 bunch spinach
- 1 cucumber
- 3 medium tomatoes
- 1 bunch celery
- 1 bunch green onions
- 3 carrots
- 1 bunch mint
- 1 bunch fresh cilantro
- 1 lime

Frozen Produce:

- 1 bag frozen peas
- 1 bag frozen spinach

Canned & Dry Goods:

- 1 can coconut milk
- 1 can black beans
- 1 can diced tomatoes
- 1 bag quinoa
- 1 bag lentils
- 1 bottle apple cider vinegar
- 1 bottle sesame oil

Nuts, Seeds & Legumes:

- 1 bag sunflower seeds
- 1 bag pumpkin seeds
- 1 bag almonds
- 1 small bag chia seeds

Dairy (or Dairy Alternatives):

- 1 container unsweetened almond milk
- 1 container coconut yogurt

Spices & Seasonings:

- Ground turmeric
- Ground coriander
- Ground cinnamon
- Ground cumin
- Himalayan pink salt
- Black pepper
- Chili flakes

Weekly Prep Instructions

To make your 30-day journey with the Pink Salt Trick Diet as efficient and stress-free as possible, batch cooking and prepping ingredients in advance can save you time and ensure you stay on track. Here's how to prep your ingredients and meals for each week:

1. Plan Your Meals for the Week

Before diving into prepping, take a few minutes to plan your meals for the week. This will help you know exactly what you need to cook, what to buy, and how to portion everything. Refer to the 30-Day Meal Plan for inspiration, or mix and match your favorite recipes from the cookbook.

Suggested Meal Prep Breakdown:

- **Breakfast:** Smoothies, Overnight Oats, Scrambled Tofu
- **Lunch:** Salads, Grain Bowls, and Stir-fries
- **Dinner:** Soups, Stews, Roasted Veggies, and Protein-rich Mains
- **Snacks:** Trail Mix, Protein Balls, Roasted Chickpeas

2. Prep Fresh Produce

a. Wash and Chop Vegetables:

Pre-wash and chop your vegetables so they're ready to use. This includes:

- Leafy greens like spinach, kale, and lettuce for salads and smoothies.
- Veggies like carrots, cucumbers, zucchini, and bell peppers for stir-fries, salads, and snacks.

- Herbs like cilantro, parsley, and mint. Store them in airtight containers with a damp paper towel to keep them fresh.

b. Roast or Cook Vegetables in Bulk:

- **Sweet Potatoes:** Peel and cube sweet potatoes, then roast them with a drizzle of olive oil and pink salt. Store them in the fridge for up to 4 days.
- **Broccoli & Cauliflower:** Cut into florets and steam or roast with olive oil and pink salt. These are great for bowls, sides, or stir-fries.

c. Pre-Cut Fruit:

- Pre-cut fruits like melon, berries, apples, or pineapple for easy access in smoothies or snacks.
- **Citrus:** Squeeze lemon and lime juice and store in a jar for quick use throughout the week.

3. Batch Cook Grains and Legumes

a. Grains:

Cook a large batch of quinoa, brown rice, or farro at the beginning of the week. These grains can be used for salads, grain bowls, or as sides for lunch and dinner.

- Store cooked grains in airtight containers in the fridge for up to 4-5 days.

b. Legumes:

If you're using canned chickpeas, black beans, or lentils, rinse and drain them.

- For dried legumes, cook them in bulk and store them in the fridge for easy access.
- Roast chickpeas with a little olive oil and your favorite spices to use as a crunchy snack.

4. Prepare Protein Sources

a. Tofu & Tempeh:

- Press tofu to remove excess moisture before using it in stir-fries, bowls, or scrambles.
- Marinate tempeh in a simple soy sauce, lemon juice, and pink salt mixture, and cook it in a stir-fry or grill it for added flavor.

b. Cook Your Lean Proteins:

- If you're using chicken or fish, cook them ahead of time in bulk, then store them in the fridge for quick additions to salads, bowls, or stir-fries.
- Boil eggs and store them in the fridge for a protein-packed snack or salad topper.

5. Prepare Sauces and Dressings

a. Salad Dressings:

Whisk together your favorite salad dressings for the week. For example, make a lemon-tahini dressing or a pink salt citrus vinaigrette.

- Store them in small mason jars or bottles for easy use throughout the week.

b. Sauces & Marinades:

Prepare soy-pink salt marinades or a pink salt tomato sauce in advance. This makes cooking meals like stir-fries or pasta dishes much quicker.

6. Assemble Snacks for the Week

a. Snack Packs:

Portion out individual servings of snacks like trail mix, roasted chickpeas, veggie sticks with hummus, or protein balls.

- Store them in small containers or snack bags, ready to grab on the go.

b. Frozen Smoothie Packs:

Assemble individual smoothie bags with your choice of frozen fruit, greens, and add-ins like chia seeds or protein powder.

- Label the bags with any additional ingredients (like coconut milk or almond milk), and keep them in the freezer for easy blending.

7. Store Everything Properly

a. Glass Jars & Containers:

Store prepped ingredients in glass containers with airtight lids to keep them fresh and organized.

- Label each container with the date you prepared the food to ensure freshness.

b. Freezer Storage:

Freeze extra portions of meals or ingredients like soups, stews, and cooked grains to keep them fresh for longer.

8. Follow a Weekly Routine

a. Meal Prep on Sundays:

Set aside 1–2 hours every Sunday to do your prep work. This is the key to staying organized and saving time throughout the week.

b. Use Leftovers Wisely:

Plan to use leftovers for lunch the next day. For example, if you make a large batch of soup or stew, you can easily reheat it for lunch or dinner.

Sample Weekly Prep Checklist:

1. **Vegetables:** Wash, chop, and roast as needed.
2. **Proteins:** Marinate, cook, and store tofu, tempeh, chicken, or fish.
3. **Grains:** Cook quinoa, rice, or farro.
4. **Legumes:** Cook or prepare canned beans and legumes.
5. **Snacks:** Assemble trail mix, roasted chickpeas, protein balls, or smoothie packs.
6. **Dressings & Sauces:** Prepare and store in mason jars or bottles.
7. **Smoothie Ingredients:** Pre-pack frozen fruits and greens

Week 1: Detox & Flush

Day	Breakfast	Lunch	Snacks	Dinner
1	Pink Salt Morning Detox Water. Avocado Toast with Pink Salt & Chili Flakes.	Grilled Chicken Salad with Pink Salt Citrus Dressing	Pink Salt Dark Chocolate Almond Bites	Lemon Garlic Salmon with Pink Salt
2	Avocado Toast with Pink Salt & Chili Flakes	Pink Salt Tuna Lettuce Wraps	Spiced Carrot Hummus with Pink Salt	Pink Salt Chicken Stir-Fry with Veggies
3	Pink Salt Veggie Omelette	Roasted Veggie & Quinoa Bowl with Pink Salt	Pink Salt Sweet Potato Chips	Vegan Cauliflower & Chickpea Curry
4	Greek Yogurt Parfait with Pink Salted Granola	Chickpea Salad with Cucumber, Dill & Pink Salt	Pink Salt Nut & Seed Trail Mix	Baked Pink Salted Cod with Citrus Zest
5	Chia Pudding with Pink Salted Mango	Zesty Pink Salt Shrimp Stir-Fry	Detox Smoothie with Cucumber, Mint & Pink Salt	Stir-Fried Tofu and Broccoli in Pink Salt Sauce
6	Almond Butter Pink Salt Smoothie	Grilled Halloumi Wraps with Pink Salted Greens	Pink Salt Edamame Pods	Grilled Eggplant with Pink Salt Herb Drizzle
7	Protein Pancakes with Pink Salted Berries	Sweet Potato & Black Bean Tacos with Pink Salt	Almond-Coconut Balls with a Pink Salt Twist	Sautéed Spinach & Mushrooms with Pink Salt

▶ Week 2: Fat Burn & Stabilize

Day	Breakfast	Lunch	Snacks	Dinner
8	Pink Salt Morning Detox Water. Overnight Oats with Himalayan Sea Salt & Figs.	Pink Salted Kale and Avocado Rice Bowl	Protein Bars with Pink Salt & Cranberries	Zucchini Noodles with Pink Salt Tomato Sauce
9	Breakfast Quinoa Bowl with Banana and Pink Salt	Baked Falafel with Pink Salt & Tahini Sauce	Pink Salt Watermelon & Mint Salad	Pink Salt Chili Lime Chicken Skewers
10	Tofu Scramble with Pink Salt	Mushroom and Pink Salt Risotto	Spicy Pink Salt Roasted Chickpeas	Stuffed Zucchini Boats with Pink Salt
11	Cinnamon-Spiced Apple Bake with Pink Salt	Pink Salt Marinated Grilled Tofu Bowl	Strawberry Coconut Shake with Pink Salt	Moroccan Chickpea Stew with Pink Salt
12	Blueberry Protein Shake with Pink Salt	Asian Slaw with Pink Salt Sesame Dressing	Green Smoothie with Lemon & Pink Salt	Thai-Inspired Pink Salt Coconut Soup
13	Pink Salt & Turmeric Coconut Milk	Roasted Seaweed Snack with Pink Salt	Frozen Banana Bites with Pink Salt & Cocoa	Teriyaki Glazed Tempeh with Pink Salt
14	Gluten-Free Breakfast Muffins with a Pink Salt Twist	Roasted Veggie & Quinoa Bowl with Pink Salt	Pink Salt Dark Chocolate Almond Bites	Lemon Garlic Salmon with Pink Salt

Week 3: Metabolism Boost

Day	Breakfast	Lunch	Snacks	Dinner
15	Pink Salt Morning Detox Water Avocado Toast with Pink Salt & Chili Flakes	Grilled Chicken Salad with Pink Salt Citrus Dressing	Spiced Carrot Hummus with Pink Salt	Vegan Cauliflower & Chickpea Curry
16	Avocado Toast with Pink Salt & Chili Flakes	Pink Salt Tuna Lettuce Wraps	Pink Salt Nut & Seed Trail Mix	Grilled Eggplant with Pink Salt Herb Drizzle
17	Pink Salt Veggie Omelette	Roasted Veggie & Quinoa Bowl with Pink Salt	Protein Bars with Pink Salt & Cranberries	Pink Salt Chicken Stir-Fry with Veggies
18	Greek Yogurt Parfait with Pink Salted Granola	Chickpea Salad with Cucumber, Dill & Pink Salt	Pink Salt Sweet Potato Chips	Stir-Fried Tofu and Broccoli in Pink Salt Sauce
19	Chia Pudding with Pink Salted Mango	Zesty Pink Salt Shrimp Stir-Fry	Detox Smoothie with Cucumber, Mint & Pink Salt	Sautéed Spinach & Mushrooms with Pink Salt
20	Almond Butter Pink Salt Smoothie	Grilled Halloumi Wraps with Pink Salted Greens	Pink Salt Watermelon & Mint Salad	Lemon Garlic Salmon with Pink Salt
21	Protein Pancakes with Pink Salted Berries	Sweet Potato & Black Bean Tacos with Pink Salt	Almond-Coconut Balls with a Pink Salt Twist	Baked Pink Salted Cod with Citrus Zest

Week 4: Tone & Sustain

Day	Breakfast	Lunch	Snacks	Dinner
22	Pink Salt Morning Detox Water. Overnight Oats with Himalayan Sea Salt & Figs.	Pink Salted Kale and Avocado Rice Bowl	Pink Salt Dark Chocolate Almond Bites	Stuffed Zucchini Boats with Pink Salt
23	Breakfast Quinoa Bowl with Banana and Pink Salt	Baked Falafel with Pink Salt & Tahini Sauce	Spicy Pink Salt Roasted Chickpeas	Moroccan Chickpea Stew with Pink Salt
24	Tofu Scramble with Pink Salt	Mushroom and Pink Salt Risotto	Pink Salt Nut & Seed Trail Mix	Pink Salt Chili Lime Chicken Skewers
25	Cinnamon-Spiced Apple Bake with Pink Salt	Pink Salt Marinated Grilled Tofu Bowl	Green Smoothie with Lemon & Pink Salt	Thai-Inspired Pink Salt Coconut Soup
26	Blueberry Protein Shake with Pink Salt	Asian Slaw with Pink Salt Sesame Dressing	Frozen Banana Bites with Pink Salt & Cocoa	Teriyaki Glazed Tempeh with Pink Salt
27	Pink Salt & Turmeric Coconut Milk	Roasted Seaweed Snack with Pink Salt	Protein Bars with Pink Salt & Cranberries	Grilled Eggplant with Pink Salt Herb Drizzle
28	Gluten-Free Breakfast Muffins with a Pink Salt Twist	Roasted Veggie & Quinoa Bowl with Pink Salt	Pink Salt Sweet Potato Chips	Pink Salt Chicken Stir-Fry with Veggies
29	Zucchini Hash with Poached Egg and Pink Salt	Grilled Chicken Salad with Pink Salt Citrus Dressing	Spiced Carrot Hummus with Pink Salt	Vegan Cauliflower & Chickpea Curry
30	Avocado Toast with Pink Salt & Chili Flakes	Pink Salt Tuna Lettuce Wraps	Pink Salt Dark Chocolate Almond Bites	Lemon Garlic Salmon with Pink Salt

CHAPTER 8: EXPERT TIPS FOR LONG-TERM SUCCESS

Avoiding Plateaus: When Progress Slows

It's common to experience periods where your progress seems to slow down or even come to a halt. This is known as a plateau, and while it can be frustrating, it's important to remember that plateaus are a natural part of the weight loss and wellness process. Understanding why plateaus happen and how to navigate through them will keep you on track and motivated to continue your journey.

What is a Plateau?

A plateau occurs when your body adapts to a particular routine, and as a result, your weight loss, detox, or metabolic improvements seem to stall. It's your body's way of saying that it has adjusted to the changes you've made, and it's time to take the next step to continue progressing.

You might experience:

- Slower weight loss despite sticking to the plan.
- No change in body measurements even though you're eating healthy.
- Reduced energy levels and heightened cravings.

These plateaus are often temporary and can be overcome by tweaking your routine, making adjustments to your diet, or shifting your exercise plan.

Why Plateaus Happen

1. Your Body Has Adapted:

When you lose weight or shift to a new diet, your metabolism may slow down as your body adjusts to a lower body mass. This can lead to slower calorie burn, meaning your progress slows even though you're doing everything right.

2. Caloric Intake vs. Expenditure:

Over time, your caloric needs may decrease as you lose weight, which can lead to a plateau if you're still eating the same number of calories. You may need to adjust your food intake or increase your physical activity to maintain a caloric deficit.

3. Hormonal Changes:

Diet changes, stress, and other lifestyle factors can lead to hormonal fluctuations that affect your metabolism. For example, leptin, the hormone responsible for regulating hunger, may decrease as you lose weight, making you feel hungrier and less satisfied.

4. Loss of Muscle Mass:

If you're not incorporating enough strength training or protein into your diet, you might lose muscle mass along with fat. This could lead to a slower metabolism since muscle burns more calories at rest than fat.

How to Overcome a Plateau

1. Track and Adjust Your Caloric Intake:

- **Recalculate Your Daily Caloric Needs:** As you lose weight, your Total Daily Energy Expenditure (TDEE) decreases. Recalculate your TDEE after a few weeks to see if you need to adjust your calorie intake.
- **Portion Control:** Even healthy foods can contribute to weight gain if portion sizes are too large. Focus on mindful eating to ensure you're eating the right amount for your goals.

2. Change Up Your Exercise Routine:

- **Add Strength Training:** If you're only doing cardio, add some resistance training or strength workouts. Building muscle increases your metabolism and helps you break through a plateau.
- **Vary Your Cardio:** Try changing the type or intensity of your cardio workouts. Switch from steady-state cardio (like walking or jogging) to interval training (HIIT) to challenge your body in new ways.
- **Increase Your Activity:** Aim for 10,000 steps a day or add a little extra movement throughout the day, like stretching, walking, or doing an additional workout.

3. Reevaluate Your Macros:

- **Increase Protein:** Protein helps to build muscle, increase satiety, and boost metabolism. If you're not already, aim to get 20-30% of your daily calories from protein.
- **Healthy Fats for Satiety:** Ensure you're getting enough healthy fats from sources like avocado, olive oil, nuts, and seeds. Healthy fats can help balance hormones, support your metabolism, and keep you feeling satisfied.
- **Monitor Carbs:** While the Pink Salt Trick Diet isn't low-carb, you might benefit from reducing your intake of refined carbs and focusing on complex carbs like whole grains and vegetables to stabilize blood sugar levels.

4. Prioritize Sleep and Stress Management:

- **Get Enough Rest:** Sleep is crucial for metabolism regulation, recovery, and weight loss. Aim for 7–9 hours of quality sleep each night. Poor sleep can lead to higher cortisol levels, making it harder to lose weight.
- **Manage Stress:** High levels of stress lead to increased cortisol production, which can affect your ability to lose weight. Practice relaxation techniques like yoga, meditation, or deep breathing exercises to reduce stress.

5. Experiment with Intermittent Fasting (IF):

- **Try IF:** If you've been following a consistent eating window, try experimenting with intermittent fasting (e.g., 16:8) to give your body a new challenge. Intermittent fasting can promote fat loss and give your digestive system a break.
- **Stay Hydrated:** Make sure you're drinking plenty of water throughout your fasting period to stay hydrated and support your body's detox process.

6. Stay Consistent and Patient:

- **Stay Consistent:** Plateaus are a normal part of any weight loss or health journey. Continue to follow the Pink Salt Trick Diet, stay active, and be patient with your progress.

- **Track Progress Differently:** Sometimes the scale doesn't reflect the changes happening in your body. Use other methods of tracking progress like measurements, clothing fit, or how you feel in terms of energy levels and mental clarity.

When to Seek Help

If you've tried several adjustments and the plateau continues for several weeks, it might be helpful to seek advice from a nutritionist, dietitian, or fitness coach who can help further personalize your plan. Sometimes a health professional can identify underlying factors like thyroid imbalances, nutritional deficiencies, or stress-related issues that could be impacting your progress.

Final Thoughts on Overcoming Plateaus

- **Stay Calm:** Plateaus are temporary, and with the right strategies, you can continue making progress.
- **Adjust, Don't Quit:** Remember that a plateau is not a reason to give up, but a signal that your body needs a slight change. Adjust your routine, try new things, and stay consistent.
- **Celebrate Non-Scale Victories:** Focus on non-scale victories such as improved energy, better sleep, or improved strength. These small wins are just as important as weight loss and contribute to overall wellness.

Adapting the Pink Salt Trick After 30 Days

Congratulations on completing the first 30 days of the Pink Salt Trick Diet! You've likely experienced significant changes in your body—whether it's weight loss, increased energy, or improved metabolism. Now that the initial phase is behind you, it's time to adapt the diet for long-term success. This next phase is all about sustaining your results, fine-tuning your routine, and maintaining a balanced lifestyle that works for you.

1. Review Your Results

Before making any changes, take a moment to assess where you are after 30 days. This reflection will help guide your next steps.

Ask Yourself:

- Have you lost weight or inches?
- Are you feeling more energized throughout the day?
- How has your digestion improved?
- Have you noticed any changes in cravings or appetite?

By reviewing these key areas, you can adjust your routine based on what's working best for your body and lifestyle.

2. Adjust Your Caloric Intake

After 30 days, your body may have adapted to your previous eating habits, and your caloric needs may have changed. This is a great time to recalculate your caloric needs to avoid hitting another plateau.

What to Do:

- Recalculate your Total Daily Energy Expenditure (TDEE) based on your current weight and activity level. As you lose weight or become more active, your caloric requirements may change.
- Adjust your caloric intake to ensure you're still in a slight deficit for continued fat loss or adjust to a maintenance level if you are happy with your results.
- **Adjust Portion Sizes:** If you're no longer aiming for weight loss, you can increase portions of healthy carbs and fats to find a maintaining balance.

3. Focus on Sustainability

While the first 30 days of the Pink Salt Trick Diet may have been about detoxing and jump-starting your weight loss, now is the time to focus on sustainability. The goal is to make this diet a long-term lifestyle, not a quick fix.

How to Sustain:

- **Stick to Whole Foods:** Continue prioritizing whole, unprocessed foods that nourish your body. Keep focusing on lean proteins, healthy fats, and fiber-rich carbohydrates.
- **Experiment with Flexibility:** Allow some flexibility in your meals. You don't need to follow the diet rigidly, but ensure that you are making healthy choices most of the time.
- **Practice Mindful Eating:** Pay attention to how much you eat, listen to your hunger cues, and practice mindful eating to avoid overeating.

4. Incorporate More Variety into Your Meals

As you move beyond the initial 30 days, it's essential to add more variety to your meals to keep things exciting and prevent boredom.

Ideas for Variety:

- Explore new spices and herbs to keep meals flavorful.
- Try different protein sources like lean meats, legumes, tofu, tempeh, or seitan.
- Add more colorful fruits and vegetables to your plate to get a variety of nutrients.
- Experiment with different cooking techniques such as grilling, steaming, or roasting to mix things up.

5. Revisit Exercise & Physical Activity

As you continue with the Pink Salt Trick Diet, maintaining an active lifestyle is key to preserving your metabolism and muscle mass.

How to Adapt Exercise:

- **Strength Training:** Incorporating strength training 2-3 times a week can help preserve muscle mass and prevent your metabolism from slowing down as you lose weight.
- **Increase Activity:** If you've been mainly doing light exercise, consider adding interval training or HIIT to boost fat burning.
- **Stay Consistent:** Keep up with regular physical activity to maintain your results. Aim for 30–60 minutes of exercise most days of the week, mixing strength training, cardio, and flexibility exercises.

6. Fine-Tune Macronutrient Ratios

As your body becomes more accustomed to the diet, it may be time to fine-tune your macronutrient ratios to better support your long-term goals.

How to Fine-Tune:

- **Protein:** Continue consuming high-quality sources of protein to maintain muscle mass and promote satiety. Aim for at least 20-30% of your total daily calories from protein-rich foods like legumes, lean meats, tofu, and quinoa.
- **Healthy Fats:** Keep your intake of healthy fats (like avocado, olive oil, and nuts) at about 25-35% of your daily calories. These fats are crucial for hormone balance, brain health, and sustained energy.
- **Carbohydrates:** Focus on complex carbs like whole grains, sweet potatoes, and vegetables for fiber and long-lasting energy. Keep your carbohydrate intake at about 40-50% of your total calories.

7. Continue Monitoring Your Progress

The journey doesn't stop after 30 days. Continue to track your progress through regular check-ins with yourself. This helps you stay accountable and make any necessary adjustments.

Ways to Monitor Progress:

- **Track Body Measurements:** Instead of focusing solely on the scale, take regular body measurements to track changes in your waist, hips, and thighs.
- **Journal Your Feelings:** Keep a food and mood journal to reflect on how certain foods make you feel and whether they support your goals.
- **Notice Non-Scale Victories:** Celebrate improvements in energy, digestion, skin health, and overall well-being, not just weight loss.

8. Maintain a Healthy Mindset

- **Be Kind to Yourself:** It's important to maintain a positive mindset throughout this process. There may be days when you don't feel at your best, and that's okay! The goal is progress, not perfection.
- **Stay Motivated:** Find new reasons to stay motivated, such as improving your physical performance, maintaining your energy levels, or working on long-term health goals.
- **Focus on Holistic Health:** Remember, this diet is not just about weight loss. It's about overall wellness, including mental, emotional, and physical health.

Making It a Lifestyle, Not a Phase

Adopting the Pink Salt Trick Diet is about more than just following a temporary plan—it's about creating lasting habits that support a healthier, more vibrant life. To truly reap the benefits of the diet and maintain your progress, it's essential to shift your mindset and embrace this as a lifestyle change, not a short-term fix.

Here are practical tips to help you make the Pink Salt Trick Diet a sustainable lifestyle that fits into your everyday routine.

1. Shift Your Mindset from "Diet" to "Lifestyle"

The first step to long-term success is to stop thinking of the Pink Salt Trick Diet as a restrictive diet plan and start seeing it as a holistic approach to wellness. This shift allows you to make healthier food choices, prioritize nutrient-dense meals, and appreciate the positive changes happening in your body.

How to Do This:

- Focus on nourishment, not restriction. Instead of focusing on what you can't eat, celebrate the nutrient-rich foods you can enjoy.
- Be patient. Understand that sustainable change takes time. Consistency is key, and small adjustments over time will lead to lasting habits.

2. Make Healthy Eating Convenient

One of the challenges people face when adopting a new eating plan is finding ways to make healthy eating convenient. After the first 30 days, you'll likely feel more comfortable with the diet's principles. To maintain your progress, make sure you have easy access to healthy meals and snacks at all times.

How to Do This:

- **Meal Prep Weekly:** Set aside time each week to prep meals and snacks. This will save you time and prevent the temptation of unhealthy, last-minute choices.
- **Stock Your Pantry:** Keep healthy staples like whole grains, legumes, nuts, seeds, and canned vegetables on hand so you can quickly throw together balanced meals.
- **Create a Go-To Snack List:** Have a list of quick, healthy snacks (like pink salt edamame pods, almond-coconut balls, or Greek yogurt parfaits) that you can grab when hunger strikes.

3. Stay Active and Engaged

Physical activity is essential for maintaining the results of the Pink Salt Trick Diet and supporting long-term health. As you continue with the plan, ensure that you're integrating regular movement into your routine to complement your nutrition and sustain your progress.

How to Do This:

- **Find a Routine That You Enjoy:** Whether it's walking, yoga, strength training, or cycling, find activities you love that will make you feel motivated and energized.
- **Make Movement a Daily Habit:** Aim for at least 30 minutes of movement each day. This can be as simple as a brisk walk, stretching after work, or a fun dance class.
- **Set Goals:** Set fitness or movement-related goals, like completing a certain number of steps, running a specific distance, or lifting a certain weight. These goals will keep you engaged and motivated.

4. Cultivate a Positive Relationship with Food

A key component of making this diet a sustainable lifestyle is cultivating a healthy relationship with food. This means not viewing food as the enemy or constantly stressing about every meal, but instead seeing it as a source of nourishment and joy.

How to Do This:

- **Practice Mindful Eating:** Slow down and pay attention to how food makes you feel. This will help you avoid overeating and help you appreciate the flavors and textures of your meals.

- **No Guilt:** Allow yourself flexibility when needed. If you indulge in something you love, don't guilt-trip yourself. It's about balance, not perfection.
- **Enjoy the Process:** Learn to enjoy cooking and experimenting with new recipes. The more fun you have in the kitchen, the easier it will be to stick to this lifestyle.

5. Learn to Navigate Social Situations

Social situations can sometimes be challenging when you're trying to eat healthy. Whether it's going to a dinner party, attending a family gathering, or eating out at a restaurant, staying on track is important for long-term success.

How to Do This:

- **Plan Ahead:** If you know you'll be attending a social event, eat a small, nutrient-dense snack beforehand so you're not tempted to overeat unhealthy foods.
- **Choose Wisely:** At restaurants or gatherings, look for options that align with the Pink Salt Trick Diet, like grilled proteins, salads with dressing on the side, or vegetable-based dishes.
- **Communicate Your Needs:** Don't be afraid to explain your dietary preferences to friends or family. Most people will appreciate your commitment to your health and will support your choices.

6. Celebrate Progress and Set New Goals

Staying motivated is easier when you're continually celebrating your progress and setting new goals. Take time to reflect on how far you've come and reward yourself for the effort you've put into your health and wellness.

How to Do This:

- **Track Non-Scale Victories:** Celebrate things like increased energy, improved digestion, better skin, or improved strength. These are just as important as weight loss.
- **Set New Health Goals:** Whether it's focusing on increasing protein intake, trying new exercises, or experimenting with new recipes, keep your goals evolving to stay motivated.
- **Reward Yourself:** Treat yourself to something special when you hit a milestone—like a massage, new workout gear, or a fun cooking class. Rewards help keep you motivated!

7. Embrace Flexibility and Patience

The key to making the Pink Salt Trick Diet a sustainable lifestyle is understanding that flexibility and patience are essential. Life will happen, and there will be days when you don't stick to the plan perfectly—and that's okay!

How to Do This:

- **Be Flexible:** If you're traveling, at a party, or simply craving something outside the plan, allow yourself the flexibility to enjoy those moments. Just get back to your routine as soon as possible.
- **Practice Patience:** Health is a lifelong journey. Don't get discouraged by minor setbacks. Stay patient with your progress and embrace the process of becoming healthier, stronger, and more energized.

8. Find Community and Support

Surround yourself with people who support your health goals. Whether it's friends, family, or an online community, having a support system will help you stay committed to the Pink Salt Trick Diet for the long term.

How to Do This:

- **Join a Community:** Find a support group or online forum where people are following similar health and wellness plans. Sharing experiences, recipes, and tips can keep you motivated.
- **Accountability Partner:** Find someone to be your accountability partner—someone who encourages you, checks in on your progress, and celebrates your wins.

Meal Prepping for Busy Weeks

We all have busy weeks when it feels like there's no time to cook, yet sticking to your Pink Salt Trick Diet goals is still important. That's where meal prepping comes in. With a bit of advance preparation, you can ensure that you always have healthy, delicious meals ready to go, even on your busiest days.

Why Meal Prep?

- **Save Time:** With meals prepped ahead of time, you won't have to spend long hours in the kitchen.
- **Stay Consistent:** Having meals ready means you're less likely to resort to unhealthy options.
- **Less Stress:** Knowing you have healthy food on hand reduces decision fatigue and saves mental energy.
- **Portion Control:** Prepping your meals helps with portion control and ensures you're eating balanced meals.

1. Plan Your Week

Before you start prepping, it's essential to plan your meals for the week. This will help you stay organized and ensure that you have all the ingredients you need.

How to Do This:

- **Choose Your Recipes:** Pick 4-5 breakfast, lunch, and dinner recipes for the week. Make sure these meals align with your goals and are easy to prepare.
- **Simplify Snacks:** Choose 2-3 snacks that are easy to make in bulk, like Pink Salted Dark Chocolate Almond Bites or Spicy Pink Salt Roasted Chickpeas.
- **Plan for Leftovers:** Cook larger portions for dinner that can be eaten for lunch the next day.
- **Create a Shopping List:** Based on your meal plan, make a detailed shopping list to ensure you have everything you need.

2. Batch Cooking: Cook in Bulk

Batch cooking is the key to efficient meal prep. Cook your grains, legumes, proteins, and vegetables in larger quantities to use throughout the week.

What to Cook in Bulk:

- **Grains:** Cook large batches of quinoa, brown rice, or farro. Store them in airtight containers for up to 4-5 days.
- **Legumes:** If you're using beans or lentils, cook them in bulk. They can be added to salads, soups, or bowls throughout the week.
- **Proteins:** Grill or bake chicken, fish, tofu, or tempeh in bulk. Store in separate containers for easy access.

- **Roasted Vegetables:** Roasting veggies like sweet potatoes, zucchini, and broccoli is an easy way to prep healthy sides for the week.

Examples of Batch Cooking:

- **Sweet Potato & Black Bean Tacos:** Roast a large tray of sweet potatoes and cook black beans in advance for a quick meal.
- **Grilled Chicken Salad:** Grill extra chicken on Sunday, and use it for lunches or dinners throughout the week.

3. Prep Snacks in Advance

Snacks are often the easiest meal to skip or replace with unhealthy options. By preparing your snacks ahead of time, you'll always have something nutritious to reach for when hunger strikes.

Snack Ideas to Prep:

- **Trail Mix:** Make a batch of Pink Salt Nut & Seed Trail Mix by combining almonds, sunflower seeds, and dried cranberries.
- **Protein Balls:** Prepare Protein Bars with Pink Salt & Cranberries or Almond-Coconut Balls with a Pink Salt Twist in advance.
- **Roasted Chickpeas:** Roast a large batch of Spicy Pink Salt Roasted Chickpeas and store them in a jar for an easy snack.
- **Pre-Cut Veggies:** Chop cucumbers, carrots, celery, and bell peppers, and store them in containers for easy snacking with hummus.

4. Prepare Breakfasts Ahead of Time

Breakfast is often the meal that gets skipped during busy mornings, but meal prepping breakfast makes it much easier to stay on track.

Breakfast Prep Ideas:

- **Overnight Oats:** Make a few jars of Overnight Oats with Himalayan Sea Salt & Figs at the beginning of the week. Add toppings like fresh fruit and nuts in the morning.
- **Chia Pudding:** Prepare Chia Pudding with Pink Salted Mango in individual servings to grab and go.
- **Smoothie Packs:** Pre-assemble Almond Butter Pink Salt Smoothie or Green Smoothie with Lemon & Pink Salt packs by adding frozen fruits, greens, and seeds to freezer bags. Just blend with liquid when you're ready.
- **Protein Pancakes:** Make a large batch of Protein Pancakes with Pink Salted Berries and freeze them. Reheat them in the microwave or toaster for a quick breakfast.

5. Store Your Meals Properly

Proper storage is essential for maintaining the quality and freshness of your prepped meals. Use clear containers so you can easily see what's inside and label them with the date they were prepared.

Storage Tips:

- **Glass Containers:** Use glass containers for storing cooked grains, legumes, proteins, and prepped vegetables. Glass helps prevent leaks and keeps food fresh for longer.
- **Freezer Bags:** Use freezer bags for storing smoothie packs, roasted veggies, and pre-portioned snacks. These can be stored in the freezer for a longer shelf life.
- **Mason Jars:** Mason jars are perfect for overnight oats, parfaits, or even salads. They keep

ingredients fresh and are easy to grab when you're on the go.

6. Simple Meal Assembly

Meal prep doesn't have to mean cooking everything from scratch. Sometimes, assembling already-prepped ingredients is all you need for a quick, satisfying meal.

Meal Assembly Ideas:

- **Bowl Meals:** Use your cooked grains, proteins, and veggies to build nourishing bowls. For example, combine roasted sweet potatoes, chickpeas, and greens, then top with Pink Salted Tahini Dressing.
- **Salads:** Keep your prepped ingredients ready for assembling salads. Add protein (tofu, chicken, or tempeh), grains, greens, and a simple dressing.
- **Wraps & Lettuce Cups:** Use lettuce leaves or gluten-free wraps and fill them with prepped proteins, veggies, and a drizzle of dressing.

7. Reheat Smartly

When it comes time to eat, it's important to reheat your meals properly. Use a stovetop, microwave, or oven depending on the meal.

- **Stovetop:** Reheat stir-fries, grains, and soups on low heat to prevent them from drying out. Add a splash of water or broth to maintain moisture.
- **Microwave:** For quick reheating, use a microwave-safe container and cover your food to retain moisture.
- **Oven:** Roasted veggies or baked proteins can be reheated in the oven at a low temperature (around 300°F) for 10-15 minutes to keep them crispy.

8. Stay Flexible with Your Plan

Even with meal prepping, there will be days when things don't go according to plan. It's important to stay flexible and not stress about it. If you have to eat out or grab something quick, aim to make healthy choices by sticking with the principles of the Pink Salt Trick Diet: whole, nutrient-dense foods with minimal processing.

Final Tips for Success:

- **Keep it Simple:** Meal prep doesn't have to be elaborate. Focus on the basics—protein, veggies, and healthy carbs—and you'll be set for the week.
- **Consistency is Key:** Regularly meal prep each week so that healthy eating becomes a habit, not a chore.
- **Enjoy the Process:** Take pride in the food you prepare. Cooking healthy meals can be a fun and rewarding experience.

Pink Salt in Restaurant Eating

Eating out at restaurants can sometimes feel like a challenge when you're trying to stick to a healthy eating plan like the Pink Salt Trick Diet. But with a little preparation and mindfulness, you can enjoy dining out without straying from your goals. Pink salt can still play a big role in making smart choices while eating at restaurants, and this section will provide you with strategies for incorporating it into your dining experiences.

1. Ask for Pink Salt or Sea Salt

While many restaurants use regular table salt, you can always ask for Himalayan pink salt or sea salt as a substitute. Pink salt has a distinct flavor and mineral content, and it's a healthier alternative to regular salt, which often contains additives like iodine or anti-caking agents.

How to Do This:

- **Politely Request:** When ordering, kindly ask if the restaurant has Himalayan pink salt. Many restaurants are happy to accommodate such requests, especially when it comes to enhancing your dining experience.
- **Bring Your Own:** If you're uncertain whether the restaurant will provide pink salt, consider bringing a small pink salt shaker with you. Many people carry small salt containers or even pink salt packets when eating out.

2. Be Mindful of Sodium Intake

Even if you're using Himalayan pink salt, it's important to be mindful of total sodium intake, especially at restaurants where dishes may already contain a lot of hidden salt.

How to Do This:

- **Ask for Salt on the Side:** Many dishes are already salted during cooking. Ask your server to bring the salt on the side so you can control how much salt you add to your meal.
- **Check the Menu for Sodium Information:** Some restaurants (especially those with healthier or more transparent menu options) may list the sodium content of their dishes. This can help you choose options with lower sodium and avoid high-sodium sauces or dishes.
- **Opt for Grilled or Roasted Dishes:** Grilled, roasted, or steamed meals often contain less added salt compared to fried or pre-marinated dishes. These options allow you to control how much salt you add.

3. Choose Whole, Unprocessed Foods

The Pink Salt Trick Diet emphasizes whole, nutrient-dense foods, and this applies even when dining out. Opt for meals that are made from fresh, whole ingredients rather than processed or packaged options.

How to Do This:

- **Go for Lean Proteins:** Choose grilled or baked chicken, fish, or plant-based proteins like tofu and tempeh. Avoid heavy sauces or deep-fried options that often contain extra fats and sodium.
- **Fresh Vegetables:** Look for dishes that include plenty of fresh, steamed, or roasted vegetables. Ask for the dressing or sauce to be served on the side to control how much is added.
- **Salads:** Salads are a great option, but be cautious of dressings and toppings that are high in sugar or sodium. Ask for olive oil and vinegar or a simple lemon wedge instead of creamy dressings.

4. Adjusting Dishes to Fit Your Diet

While it's easy to stick to your plan when cooking at home, dining out can present some challenges. However, many restaurants are open to making adjustments to accommodate your dietary preferences.

How to Do This:

- **Request Modifications:** Don't be afraid to ask for customizations. For example, ask for a dish to be made without sauces or to have it grilled instead of fried.

- **Choose Simpler Options:** If a dish comes with heavy sauces or seasonings, ask for it to be made plain or with light seasoning, and then add your own Himalayan pink salt at the table.
- **Request Steamed or Grilled:** Many restaurant meals are sautéed or fried in butter or oils. Opt for steamed, grilled, or broiled versions instead, which are typically healthier.

5. Smart Drink Choices

When it comes to beverages, it's just as important to make mindful choices. Soft drinks, sugary juices, and alcohol can sometimes derail your progress.

How to Do This:

- **Water:** Stick with still or sparkling water. You can add a splash of lemon for extra flavor or request your water with pink salt if you prefer. It's a great way to get your electrolytes while keeping your sodium intake balanced.
- **Herbal Teas:** Opt for unsweetened herbal teas like ginger, peppermint, or chamomile to aid digestion without extra sugar.
- **Limit Sugary Drinks:** Avoid sugary sodas or fruit juices. These can spike your blood sugar and lead to cravings.
- **Alcohol:** If you choose to drink, opt for a glass of wine or a clear spirit like vodka or gin with a low-calorie mixer. Avoid sugary cocktails and large mixed drinks.

6. Choose Simpler Desserts or Skip Them

Desserts are often loaded with sugar, artificial additives, and excess calories. Instead of indulging in calorie-heavy treats, consider a simpler, more natural dessert.

How to Do This:

- **Fruit-Based Desserts:** Look for desserts that feature fresh fruit, like grilled peaches or a fruit salad. These options are naturally sweet and full of nutrients.
- **Skip the Dessert:** If you're not in the mood for a sweet treat, skip dessert altogether or ask for a small portion of something light like fresh berries or a small piece of dark chocolate.
- **Bring Your Own Dessert:** In some cases, you can bring your own healthy homemade dessert, like Pink Salt Dark Chocolate Almond Bites, to enjoy after your meal.

7. Stay Consistent While Dining Out

It's perfectly fine to enjoy eating out while following the Pink Salt Trick Diet, but it's important to stay consistent with the principles of the diet. This means making healthy choices that support your overall wellness goals without feeling deprived or stressed.

How to Do This:

- **Stay on Track:** If you indulge in a heavier meal at one restaurant, balance it out with lighter meals the next day or opt for lighter dishes the following meal.
- **Portion Control:** Restaurant portions tend to be large, so consider sharing dishes or asking for a to-go box and saving half for later.
- **Practice Gratitude:** Be mindful of the experience. Appreciate the food, the company, and the enjoyment of eating out without overindulging.

Final Thoughts on Eating Out

Dining out doesn't have to derail your progress on the Pink Salt Trick Diet. With a little planning, asking for modifications, and making mindful choices, you can continue to enjoy eating out without compromising your health goals. Always remember, it's about balance, flexibility, and making smart choices that align with your wellness journey.

Staying Motivated & Measuring Progress

Staying motivated throughout your wellness journey can be challenging, especially when progress seems slow or when life gets busy. However, maintaining focus on your long-term health goals is key to staying on track with the Pink Salt Trick Diet. Equally important is measuring your progress—both to celebrate victories and to make adjustments when necessary. Here's how you can stay motivated and measure your progress effectively.

1. Set Clear and Realistic Goals

To stay motivated, it's crucial to have clear goals that guide your journey. Having a sense of direction helps you stay on track and reminds you why you started.

How to Set Effective Goals:

a. Be Specific: Instead of vague goals like "lose weight," aim for more specific targets like "lose 5 pounds in 4 weeks" or "reduce my waist measurement by 2 inches."

b. Make Them Achievable: Ensure your goals are realistic. Setting overly ambitious goals may lead to disappointment if they're not reached in the short term.

c. Set Long-Term and Short-Term Goals:

- **Long-Term Goals:** These are the bigger picture, such as "achieve a healthy weight" or "increase energy and fitness."
- **Short-Term Goals:** These keep you motivated in the immediate term, like "meal prep for the week" or "complete 3 strength training sessions this week."

2. Track Your Progress in Different Ways

Measuring progress goes beyond just looking at the scale. There are multiple ways to track your success—some of which may be more meaningful than the number on the scale.

Ways to Track Your Progress:

- **Take Photos:** Take progress photos at regular intervals (e.g., weekly or bi-weekly). These photos can provide a more visual representation of changes in your body composition that the scale might not show.
- **Use a Tape Measure:** Track changes in your waist, hips, thighs, and arms using a measuring tape. Sometimes, you might be losing inches even if your weight stays the same.
- **Track Fitness Gains:** Keep a record of your physical performance, such as how much weight you're lifting, how fast or far you can run, or your flexibility. Progress in fitness is a great indicator of health improvements.
- **Journal How You Feel:** Record how you feel each day in terms of energy, mood, sleep quality, and digestion. These subjective measures can highlight the internal benefits of your diet and wellness routine.

3. Celebrate Non-Scale Victories

Weight is not the only way to measure success. Non-scale victories (NSVs) can be just as important—and often more meaningful. When you celebrate these victories, you'll stay motivated and appreciate the positive changes in your life.

Examples of Non-Scale Victories:

- **Increased Energy:** You're feeling more energized throughout the day and not relying on caffeine.
- **Improved Sleep:** You're sleeping more soundly and waking up feeling rested.
- **Better Digestion:** You've noticed fewer bloating episodes, improved gut health, or more regular digestion.
- **Clothing Fit:** Your clothes fit more comfortably, or you're fitting into clothes that were previously too tight.
- **Increased Strength or Endurance:** You're lifting heavier weights, running longer distances, or feeling stronger and more capable during workouts.

4. Stay Accountable

Accountability can make a huge difference in staying motivated. Having someone to check in with helps ensure that you stay consistent and committed to your goals.

Ways to Stay Accountable:

- **Find an Accountability Partner:** This could be a friend, family member, or even someone online who is also following the Pink Salt Trick Diet or a similar plan. Set regular check-ins to discuss progress, share challenges, and motivate each other.
- **Join Online Communities:** Many online groups, forums, or social media groups are centered around health and wellness goals. You can find support, share progress, and get encouragement from others on similar journeys.
- **Track Your Progress in an App or Journal:** Using apps like MyFitnessPal or Lose It! to log meals, exercise, and goals can keep you accountable and help you stay on track.

5. Stay Flexible and Adjust When Necessary

It's important to stay flexible in your approach. Life happens, and there will be times when you need to adjust your routine. Whether it's due to a busy week, a holiday, or a slip-up, don't get discouraged. Adjustments are part of the process, and as long as you stay committed, progress will come.

How to Adapt When Needed:

- **If Progress Slows:** If you find that your progress has stalled (a common occurrence after a few weeks), it may be time to adjust your calorie intake, switch up your exercise routine, or tweak your macronutrient balance. Consider incorporating more strength training or reducing processed foods to shake things up.
- **If Life Gets in the Way:** If you miss a workout or have an off-track day, simply get back on the wagon the next day. One missed workout or indulgence isn't going to undo all your progress. Stay patient and focus on the long-term benefits.
- **Celebrate Imperfection:** Perfection isn't the goal. It's about consistency. Don't be too hard on

yourself for occasional slip-ups. Progress is made through small, consistent efforts over time.

6. Focus on the Bigger Picture

While the diet and exercise changes you're making are important, it's also vital to keep in mind that the ultimate goal is to create sustainable health habits that will last for life. By shifting your focus from quick fixes to long-term wellness, you'll be able to stay motivated and committed to the lifestyle changes you're making.

How to Focus on the Bigger Picture:

- **Mindset Shift:** View this journey as a lifestyle change, not a short-term fix. Your goal is not just to lose weight but to improve overall health, build habits, and feel your best every day.
- **Enjoy the Process:** Embrace the journey, not just the destination. Find joy in cooking new meals, trying new workouts, and learning about your body's needs. Celebrate the milestones along the way!

7. Reflect and Re-Evaluate Regularly

Regularly reflecting on your goals and progress helps keep your motivation high and ensures that you're always moving forward. This reflection process also provides an opportunity to re-evaluate your goals and make adjustments to your plan if necessary.

How to Reflect & Re-Evaluate:

- **Monthly Check-ins:** At the end of each month, take some time to reflect on how far you've come. Write down what's working, what's challenging, and any insights you've gained. Use this as an opportunity to adjust your goals or strategies for the next month.
- **Celebrate Milestones:** Whether you've lost 5 pounds, completed a challenging workout, or stuck to your meal plan for a month, celebrate these milestones! Take time to appreciate your hard work and use that motivation to propel you forward.

CHAPTER 9: FREQUENTLY ASKED QUESTIONS

> **Can I use pink salt if I have high blood pressure?**

The short answer is yes, but with important considerations. Here's an in-depth look at Himalayan pink salt and its impact on high blood pressure:

Pink Salt vs. Regular Table Salt

Himalayan pink salt is often touted as a healthier alternative to regular table salt because it contains a variety of minerals, including magnesium, potassium, calcium, and iron. These trace minerals can provide small health benefits, but the sodium content in pink salt is similar to table salt, which can still have an impact on blood pressure if consumed in excess.

How Sodium Affects High Blood Pressure

The main concern for individuals with high blood pressure (hypertension) is sodium intake. Sodium causes the body to retain more fluid, which can increase the volume of blood circulating in your system. This added volume can lead to higher blood pressure. Whether it's from pink salt or regular salt, too much sodium can exacerbate hypertension.

How Much Sodium Is Too Much?

The American Heart Association (AHA) recommends that adults limit their sodium intake to no more than 2,300 milligrams per day, and ideally aim for 1,500 milligrams for those with high blood pressure. This amount is equivalent to 1 teaspoon of regular table salt or Himalayan pink salt.

If you have high blood pressure, it's essential to monitor your total sodium intake throughout the day, including all food sources (processed foods, restaurant meals, condiments, etc.), and not just what you add to your food.

Benefits of Pink Salt for High Blood Pressure

While pink salt contains trace minerals like potassium, which can help counterbalance the effects of sodium and potentially support heart health, the amount of potassium in pink salt is quite small compared to foods naturally rich in potassium (such as bananas, sweet potatoes, and leafy greens). Therefore, relying solely on pink salt for potassium benefits may not have a significant effect on blood pressure.

Additionally, pink salt doesn't have the additives found in regular table salt, such as anti-caking agents, which can sometimes cause inflammation in the body. However, this benefit is more of a minor consideration in terms of high blood pressure.

How to Use Pink Salt Safely if You Have High Blood Pressure

If you decide to use Himalayan pink salt, consider these tips for managing your blood pressure:

1. Limit Salt Usage: Even though pink salt is a more natural alternative, it still contains sodium. Use it sparingly in cooking and as a finishing salt. Be mindful of the total amount of sodium in your daily diet.

2. Increase Potassium-Rich Foods: While pink salt has some potassium, you should focus on increasing potassium-rich foods like avocados, spinach, sweet potatoes, and bananas. Potassium helps balance the effects of sodium in the body and can help lower blood pressure.

3. Stay Hydrated: Adequate hydration helps the kidneys flush excess sodium out of the body. Drinking plenty of water throughout the day can help support healthy blood pressure.

4. Watch Processed Foods: Many processed and packaged foods contain high amounts of sodium, even if they don't taste salty. Avoiding these foods will help you keep your sodium intake in check.

5. Consult Your Doctor: If you have high blood pressure, it's always wise to consult your healthcare provider before making changes to your diet. They can provide personalized guidance based on your medical history.

Final Thoughts

While Himalayan pink salt may offer some benefits over regular table salt, the most important factor in managing high blood pressure is reducing sodium intake overall. Pink salt is not a free pass to add more salt to your diet, especially if you're dealing with hypertension. Use it moderately, focus on a balanced diet rich in potassium, and ensure you're staying hydrated for optimal heart health.

Will I lose weight just by adding pink salt?

Adding Himalayan pink salt to your diet alone is unlikely to result in weight loss. While pink salt offers some health benefits, such as providing essential minerals like potassium and magnesium, weight loss is a complex process that involves a combination of factors, including dietary changes, exercise, and overall calorie intake.

Here's a breakdown of why just adding pink salt won't be a magic solution for weight loss:

1. Salt and Weight Loss: What Pink Salt Does

Himalayan pink salt can have some benefits for overall health, such as:

- **Hydration:** Pink salt can help maintain electrolyte balance and support hydration by promoting proper water retention. However, water retention does not equate to fat loss.
- **Appetite Control:** There are some claims that adding a small amount of pink salt to water can help reduce cravings, but this effect is generally modest and does not significantly impact weight loss.

However, pink salt alone will not directly lead to fat burning or weight loss.

2. The Role of Sodium in the Body

While sodium (found in all salts, including pink salt) plays a crucial role in the body, too much sodium can cause water retention, which may make you feel bloated or heavier. This can give the illusion of weight gain, but it's not related to actual fat gain.

For weight loss, the focus should be on maintaining a caloric deficit—burning more calories than you consume. Simply adding salt will not create this deficit.

3. What Actually Leads to Weight Loss

To lose weight, you must create a caloric deficit, which means:

- Eating fewer calories than your body needs for maintenance or
- Increasing physical activity to burn more calories than you consume.

A healthy weight loss strategy includes:

- Consuming a balanced diet of whole foods (fruits, vegetables, lean proteins, healthy fats, whole grains).
- Exercising regularly to burn calories and increase metabolism.
- Practicing portion control and being mindful of your calorie intake.

4. Pink Salt and Detoxification

Some people claim that pink salt can help with detoxification due to its mineral content and its ability to balance electrolytes. While detoxing can support overall well-being, detoxification alone does not directly lead to weight loss. It's about creating a healthy environment for your body to function optimally.

5. Maintaining a Healthy Relationship with Salt

It's essential to use pink salt moderately and be mindful of your total sodium intake throughout the day. While it's generally healthier than table salt due to its trace minerals, it still contains sodium, which should be consumed in moderation, especially if you have high blood pressure or are sensitive to sodium.

How to Incorporate Pink Salt Into a Weight Loss Plan

While pink salt alone won't lead to weight loss, you can use it as part of a healthy eating plan:

- **Use it to season meals:** Add a pinch of pink salt to your meals to enhance flavor without adding excessive sodium.
- **Stay mindful of your sodium intake:** Avoid over-salting your food, and be mindful of other sources of sodium in processed foods.
- **Hydrate well:** Drinking water with a pinch of pink salt can support hydration and electrolyte balance, which may make you feel better and less bloated.

> **What are signs of overconsumption?**

Overconsumption of Himalayan pink salt (or any type of salt) can lead to various health issues, primarily related to sodium intake. While pink salt contains beneficial trace minerals, it still contains sodium, which, when consumed in excessive amounts, can have negative effects on your body.

Here are some signs of overconsumption of salt:

1. Water Retention and Bloating

One of the most common signs of too much sodium is water retention. When you consume excessive amounts of salt, your body retains extra fluid to balance the sodium levels, leading to bloating and puffiness.

Symptoms may include:

- Swollen ankles or feet
- Puffy face or hands
- Stomach bloating

This is because excess sodium disrupts the balance of fluids in your body, causing you to retain more water than usual.

2. High Blood Pressure (Hypertension)

Excessive sodium intake is directly linked to high blood pressure (hypertension), which can strain your heart, kidneys, and blood vessels. Over time, chronic high blood pressure can increase your risk of heart disease, stroke, and kidney damage.

Symptoms to watch for:

- Headaches (due to increased pressure on blood vessels)
- Dizziness or lightheadedness
- Shortness of breath during physical activity
- Chest pain or a feeling of pressure

If you notice any of these signs, it's important to consult a healthcare provider.

3. Increased Thirst

One of the body's natural responses to excess salt is increased thirst. If you're consuming too much sodium, your kidneys work to flush out the excess, which can lead to dehydration and cause you to feel thirsty more frequently.

Symptoms may include:

- Constant thirst
- Dry mouth
- Urination issues, such as feeling like you need to urinate more often

4. Frequent Urination

Excess sodium increases the body's need to excrete water through urination. If you're consuming too much salt, you may find yourself going to the bathroom more often to flush out the extra sodium and maintain fluid balance.

5. Headaches

Excess sodium can lead to dehydration, which in turn may cause headaches. When your body retains extra water to dilute the sodium, it can disrupt fluid balance in your brain, leading to tension headaches or migraines.

6. Kidney Strain

Your kidneys are responsible for filtering out excess sodium from your body. If you consume too much salt over an extended period, it can put a strain on your kidneys and may lead to kidney problems or even kidney disease.

Symptoms may include:

- Pain in the lower back or sides (where kidneys are located)
- Changes in urination (dark-colored urine, increased or decreased frequency)

7. Digestive Issues

Overconsumption of salt can irritate your stomach lining, leading to discomfort or digestive problems. You may experience symptoms such as:

- Stomach pain
- Acid reflux

- Indigestion
- Nausea

8. Fatigue or Weakness

Excess sodium can lead to an imbalance of electrolytes, particularly potassium and magnesium, which are necessary for proper muscle function and energy levels. This imbalance can cause you to feel fatigued or weak.

Symptoms may include:

- Low energy
- Weakness in muscles
- Tiredness that doesn't improve with rest

9. Heart Palpitations

High sodium levels can also affect your heart rate, potentially leading to irregular heartbeats or palpitations. In extreme cases, this can result in serious cardiovascular problems.

Symptoms may include:

- Feeling of rapid or irregular heartbeats
- Fluttering sensation in your chest

> Can I combine this with intermittent fasting?

Yes, you can combine the Pink Salt Trick Diet with intermittent fasting (IF), and many people find this combination effective for achieving their health and wellness goals. However, there are a few key things to consider when combining these two approaches to ensure you're optimizing your results safely and effectively.

How the Pink Salt Trick Diet and Intermittent Fasting Work Together

Both the Pink Salt Trick Diet and intermittent fasting focus on promoting better health, weight loss, and metabolism-boosting by managing your intake and timing of nutrients. Here's how they can complement each other:

1. Electrolyte Balance During Fasting

One of the challenges people face when doing intermittent fasting is maintaining electrolyte balance, especially if they're consuming fewer calories or fluids during fasting periods. Himalayan pink salt can help with this, as it's rich in minerals like sodium, potassium, calcium, and magnesium—which are essential for hydration, nerve function, and muscle contractions.

How it helps:

- Pink salt can help prevent symptoms of electrolyte imbalance during fasting, such as headaches, muscle cramps, and fatigue.
- Adding a pinch of pink salt to your water in the morning or during fasting hours helps maintain proper hydration and mineral balance, making fasting periods more comfortable.

2. Appetite Control During Fasting

Some people struggle with hunger or cravings during fasting periods, especially if they're just starting out with intermittent fasting. The Pink Salt Trick Diet has an appetite-suppressing component, as the sodium in Himalayan pink salt can help regulate appetite and cravings.

How it helps:

- Pink salt can help control hunger by supporting hydration and balancing electrolytes, which can prevent overeating when you break your fast.
- Drinking pink salt water during fasting periods can help curb cravings and make it easier to stick to your fasting window.

3. Sustainable Weight Loss

When combining intermittent fasting with the Pink Salt Trick Diet, you're focusing on foods that are whole, nutrient-dense, and mineral-rich. These qualities help support long-term weight loss and sustainable results.

How it helps:

- Pink salt does not cause weight gain when consumed moderately. It supports your metabolism and helps with detoxification, which is particularly beneficial during a fast.
- The Pink Salt Trick Diet prioritizes whole foods, which provide the energy and nutrition your body needs during eating windows, supporting healthy fat loss without feeling deprived.

4. Timing Your Salt Intake During Fasting

During fasting, it's important to maintain your electrolyte balance without disrupting your fast. Here's how you can incorporate pink salt without affecting the benefits of fasting:

How to incorporate pink salt while fasting:

- **Pink Salt Water:** You can drink water with a pinch of pink salt during fasting hours to maintain electrolytes without breaking the fast, as it contains no calories.
- **During Eating Windows:** Add pink salt to your meals during your eating windows (lunch or dinner) to enhance flavor and improve digestion.

Things to Keep in Mind:

1. Stay Hydrated: When fasting, it's essential to stay hydrated to support your metabolism, energy levels, and overall health. Drink plenty of water throughout the day, and consider adding a pinch of pink salt to your water for electrolyte balance.

2. Moderation is Key: While Himalayan pink salt is beneficial, it's still important to consume it moderately, as excessive sodium intake can negatively affect your blood pressure and kidneys over time. Stick to the recommended amount and listen to your body.

3. Balanced Meals During Eating Windows: To maximize the benefits of intermittent fasting, focus on nutrient-dense meals when you break your fast. Include a balance of protein, healthy fats, and complex carbohydrates. This will fuel your body and prevent overeating, while keeping your metabolism elevated.

4. Avoid Over-Salting: Many people tend to over-salt their food, especially during periods of fasting. Be mindful of how much pink salt you're using—just a pinch can go a long way in improving flavor and electrolyte balance.

What if I miss a day of the trick?

Missing a day of the Pink Salt Trick Diet is not a huge setback. Life happens, and skipping a day here or there won't derail your progress if you continue to follow the principles of the diet most of the time. It's important to approach your wellness journey with flexibility and patience—this is about creating lasting, healthy habits, not striving for perfection.

Here's what you can do if you miss a day of the Pink Salt Trick Diet:

1. Don't Stress, Just Get Back on Track

The most important thing to remember is that one missed day won't undo your progress. It's easy to get discouraged, but the key is getting back on track as soon as possible.

What to Do:

- Get back to your routine the next day. There's no need to "make up" for the missed day, just continue with your regular meals, hydration, and salt routine.
- **Avoid guilt:** It's perfectly normal to have a day where things don't go according to plan. Remind yourself that progress is a long-term process.

2. Hydrate Well

If you missed your Pink Salt Morning Detox Water, it's a good idea to start your next day with a fresh glass of water with pink salt. It will help rehydrate your body, replenish electrolytes, and kickstart your metabolism.

What to Do:

- Drink water with a pinch of Himalayan pink salt to restore hydration and balance electrolytes.
- Hydrate throughout the day with water, herbal teas, or infused water to support your body's natural detox process.

3. Don't Overcompensate with Salt

If you missed the pink salt one day, resist the urge to overdo it the next day. Over-consumption of salt can lead to water retention and other health issues. Stick to a moderate amount of salt, as recommended, to maintain balance.

What to Do:

- Use pink salt sparingly in your meals and drinks, following the regular guidelines, without overcompensating.

4. Focus on Nutrient-Dense Foods

If you missed your usual meals or snacks with pink salt, ensure that you focus on nutrient-dense foods for the rest of the day. This will keep your metabolism stable and help you feel your best.

What to Do:

- Include plenty of whole foods, like vegetables, lean proteins, healthy fats, and complex carbs, to keep your body nourished.
- Stay mindful of your portion sizes to ensure you're eating balanced, satisfying meals without overindulging.

5. Stay Consistent, Not Perfect

Missing one day doesn't mean you've failed. The key to success is consistency, not perfection. Life will always throw curveballs, so give yourself permission to miss a day and move forward with confidence.

What to Do:

- If you miss a day, it's okay to feel a little frustrated, but don't let it derail your entire journey. Reflect, learn from the experience, and continue.

- Consistency over time is what leads to lasting results, so keep up your efforts and focus on the bigger picture.

6. Reflect on Your Progress

Missing a day can sometimes be a good opportunity to reflect on your progress and see how far you've come. Instead of focusing on the setback, take note of the positive changes you've experienced during your time on the Pink Salt Trick Diet.

What to Do:

- Track your progress with photos, measurements, or how you're feeling. Celebrate non-scale victories, like increased energy, improved digestion, or better sleep.
- Acknowledge your dedication to making healthier choices, even if you miss a day. This positive mindset will keep you motivated moving forward.

7. Use It as a Learning Opportunity

If missing a day happens frequently or becomes a pattern, use it as an opportunity to evaluate your routine. Perhaps you need to adjust your meal prep, plan ahead for busier days, or make the diet more flexible to suit your lifestyle better.

What to Do:

- Identify triggers that lead to missing your routine. Is it a busy schedule, lack of planning, or something else? Make small changes to address these challenges.
- Adapt the plan to fit your lifestyle. The Pink Salt Trick Diet should be flexible enough to make it easy to follow, even on busy days.

CHAPTER 10: MEASUREMENT CONVERSIONS & NUTRITIONAL GUIDELINES

Metric/Imperial Conversion Charts

Volume Conversions

Metric (ml)	Imperial (fl. oz.)	Imperial (cups)	Imperial (tbsp)	Imperial (tsp)
1 ml	0.034 fl. oz.	0.004 cups	0.067 tbsp	0.202 tsp
5 ml	0.17 fl. oz.	0.02 cups	1 tbsp	1 tsp
15 ml	0.51 fl. oz.	0.063 cups	3 tbsp	3 tsp
30 ml	1.02 fl. oz.	0.125 cups	6 tbsp	6 tsp
60 ml	2.04 fl. oz.	0.25 cups	12 tbsp	12 tsp
100 ml	3.38 fl. oz.	0.42 cups	16.8 tbsp	20 tsp
250 ml	8.45 fl. oz.	1 cup	32 tbsp	60 tsp

Weight Conversions

Metric (g)	Imperial (oz.)	Imperial (lbs.)
1 g	0.035 oz.	0.0022 lbs.
5 g	0.18 oz.	0.011 lbs.
10 g	0.35 oz.	0.022 lbs.
25 g	0.88 oz.	0.055 lbs.
50 g	1.76 oz.	0.11 lbs.
100 g	3.53 oz.	0.22 lbs.
250 g	8.82 oz.	0.55 lbs.
500 g	17.64 oz.	1.1 lbs.
1 kg	35.27 oz.	2.2 lbs.

Temperature Conversions

Celsius (°C)	Fahrenheit (°F)
0°C	32°F
5°C	41°F
10°C	50°F
15°C	59°F
20°C	68°F
25°C	77°F
30°C	86°F
35°C	95°F
40°C	104°F
100°C	212°F

Portion Size Guide

Eating the right portion sizes is key to controlling calorie intake, ensuring proper nutrient balance, and achieving sustainable weight loss or maintenance. This portion size guide is designed to help you make healthy choices without overindulging.

1. Protein Sources

Protein is essential for muscle maintenance, satiety, and overall health. The following portion sizes are a good guide for different types of protein:

a. Chicken or Turkey (cooked):

- Serving Size: 3–4 ounces (about the size of a deck of cards)
- Calories: ~140–170 calories per 4 oz

b. Fish (salmon, cod, tilapia):

- Serving Size: 3–4 ounces (about the size of a deck of cards)
- Calories: ~120–200 calories per 4 oz

c. Tofu or Tempeh:

- Serving Size: 1/2 block (about 4–5 ounces)
- Calories: ~120–200 calories per 4 oz (depending on type)

d. Eggs:

- Serving Size: 2 large eggs
- Calories: ~140–160 calories for 2 eggs

e. Lean Beef (cooked):

- Serving Size: 3 ounces (about the size of a deck of cards)
- Calories: ~180–250 calories per 3 oz (depending on the cut)

f. Legumes (beans, lentils):

- Serving Size: 1/2 cup cooked
- Calories: ~100–130 calories per 1/2 cup

2. Vegetables

Vegetables are nutrient-dense and low in calories, making them perfect for filling up while maintaining a healthy weight. Here are some typical serving sizes for different types of vegetables:

a. Leafy Greens (spinach, kale, arugula):

- Serving Size: 1–2 cups raw (about the size of a baseball)
- Calories: ~7–15 calories per cup

b. Non-Starchy Vegetables (zucchini, bell peppers, broccoli):

- Serving Size: 1 cup cooked or raw
- Calories: ~20–50 calories per cup

c. Starchy Vegetables (sweet potatoes, corn, peas):

- Serving Size: 1/2 cup cooked (about the size of a small fist)
- Calories: ~80–120 calories per 1/2 cup

d. Cucumber, Celery, Carrots (raw):

- Serving Size: 1 cup raw (about the size of a fist)
- Calories: ~20–40 calories per cup

3. Grains

Grains provide carbohydrates for energy and are an important part of a balanced diet. Portion sizes help prevent overconsumption while maintaining your energy levels.

a. Quinoa, Brown Rice, Barley (cooked):

- Serving Size: 1/2 cup cooked
- Calories: ~100–120 calories per 1/2 cup

b. Oats (cooked):

- Serving Size: 1/2 cup cooked
- Calories: ~150 calories per 1/2 cup

c. Whole Wheat Pasta (cooked):

- Serving Size: 1/2 cup cooked
- Calories: ~150 calories per 1/2 cup

d. Bread (whole grain):

- Serving Size: 1 slice
- Calories: ~80–100 calories per slice

4. Healthy Fats

Fats are important for overall health and hormone balance, but they are calorie-dense, so portion control is essential.

a. Avocado:

- Serving Size: 1/4 to 1/2 avocado (about the size of a small fist)
- Calories: ~60–120 calories per 1/4 to 1/2 avocado

b. Olive Oil:

- Serving Size: 1 tablespoon
- Calories: ~120 calories per tablespoon

c. Nuts & Seeds (almonds, sunflower seeds, chia):

- Serving Size: 1 ounce (about 23 almonds or 2 tablespoons of seeds)
- Calories: ~160–200 calories per ounce

d. Nut Butters (peanut, almond, cashew):

- Serving Size: 1 tablespoon
- Calories: ~90–100 calories per tablespoon

5. Fruits

Fruits are rich in vitamins, minerals, and fiber, making them an excellent part of a balanced diet. Here are typical serving sizes for different fruits:

a. Apples, Oranges, Pears:

- Serving Size: 1 medium fruit (about the size of a tennis ball)
- Calories: ~70–100 calories per medium fruit

b. Berries (strawberries, blueberries, raspberries):

- Serving Size: 1/2 cup
- Calories: ~30–50 calories per 1/2 cup

c. Bananas:

- Serving Size: 1 medium banana
- Calories: ~100–120 calories per banana

d. Grapes:

- Serving Size: 1/2 cup (about 15 grapes)
- Calories: ~50–60 calories per 1/2 cup

6. Dairy & Dairy Alternatives

Dairy products provide calcium, protein, and other essential nutrients. If you're using dairy alternatives, be sure to choose options that are fortified with calcium and vitamin D.

a. Greek Yogurt:

- Serving Size: 1/2 cup
- Calories: ~100–120 calories per 1/2 cup

b. Milk (cow's milk or plant-based):

- Serving Size: 1 cup
- Calories: ~80–150 calories per cup (depending on type)

c. Cheese (hard cheeses like cheddar, mozzarella):

- Serving Size: 1 ounce (about the size of a pair of dice)
- Calories: ~100–120 calories per ounce

d. Cottage Cheese:

- Serving Size: 1/2 cup
- Calories: ~100–120 calories per 1/2 cup

7. Beverages

Beverages can add extra calories, especially if they contain sugar or creamer. Here's a guide for managing your drink portions:

a. Water:

- Serving Size: As needed, aim for 8 cups (about 2 liters) per day
- Calories: 0 calories

b. Coffee (black, with no added sugar or cream):

- Serving Size: 1 cup
- Calories: 0–5 calories per cup

c. Tea (unsweetened):

- Serving Size: 1 cup
- Calories: 0–5 calories per cup

d. Smoothies:

- Serving Size: 1 cup (made from whole fruits, veggies, and water or unsweetened milk)
- Calories: ~150–250 calories per cup (depending on ingredients)

General Guidelines for Portion Control

Use your hand as a guide:

- **Protein:** The size of your palm (for lean meats, fish, or tofu).
- **Carbs:** The size of your fist (for grains or starchy vegetables).
- **Fats:** The size of your thumb (for oils, nuts, or nut butters).
- **Vegetables:** The size of your two cupped hands (for leafy greens or non-starchy vegetables).

Understanding Macronutrients

Macronutrients are the three primary types of nutrients that provide energy to the body. They are essential for maintaining bodily functions, supporting metabolism, building muscle, and keeping you feeling satisfied. The three main types of macronutrients are protein, carbohydrates, and fats. Each plays a distinct role in your body, and the balance of these macronutrients is key to achieving optimal health and wellness.

1. Protein: The Building Block of Your Body

Protein is one of the most important macronutrients for muscle growth, repair, and overall cellular function. It's especially important for maintaining muscle mass when you're following a weight loss plan or engaging in regular physical activity. Protein also helps boost metabolism and promotes satiety, making you feel full longer.

Why You Need Protein:

- **Muscle repair and growth:** Protein helps repair muscle fibers after workouts and promotes muscle growth.
- **Immune function:** Proteins are essential for creating enzymes and antibodies that fight infection.
- **Satiety:** Protein helps you feel full, which can prevent overeating and assist with weight management.

Sources of Protein:

- **Animal-based:** Chicken, turkey, fish, eggs, lean beef, dairy (Greek yogurt, cheese)
- **Plant-based:** Lentils, chickpeas, quinoa, tofu, tempeh, edamame, nuts, seeds

How Much Protein Do You Need?

- **General guideline:** Aim for 0.8 to 1 gram of protein per kilogram of body weight for general health.
- **For weight loss or muscle gain:** You may need more protein, around 1.2 to 2 grams per kilogram of body weight.

2. Carbohydrates: Your Body's Primary Source of Energy

Carbohydrates are the body's preferred energy source. They are broken down into glucose (sugar) in the body, which fuels muscles and organs, including the brain. Carbs are essential for providing sustained energy for daily activities and exercise.

Why You Need Carbohydrates:

- **Energy:** Carbs are your body's primary fuel source for physical activity and basic bodily functions.
- **Brain function:** Your brain requires glucose to function, so carbs help maintain mental clarity and focus.
- **Digestive health:** Many carbohydrate-rich foods contain fiber, which promotes digestive health, regulates bowel movements, and supports gut health.

Types of Carbohydrates:

- **Simple Carbs:** Found in foods like fruit, dairy, and processed sugars (candy, pastries). Simple carbs provide quick energy but can cause blood sugar spikes and crashes if consumed in excess.
- **Complex Carbs:** Found in whole grains (brown rice, quinoa, oats), legumes (lentils, chickpeas), starchy vegetables (sweet potatoes, butternut squash), and whole fruits. These provide slow-releasing energy and are often higher in fiber.

How Much Carbohydrates Do You Need?

- **General guideline:** 45–65% of your daily calories should come from carbohydrates, depending on your activity level.
- **For weight loss:** You may opt for lower-carb diets, but make sure to focus on healthy, whole-food carbs, including vegetables, fruits, and whole grains.

3. Fats: Essential for Hormonal Balance and Energy

Fats are often misunderstood, but they are crucial for overall health. They support brain function, cell structure, hormonal regulation, and absorption of fat-soluble vitamins (A, D, E, K). Healthy fats are also an important energy source, especially during periods of low activity or when you're fasting.

Why You Need Fats:

- **Energy storage:** Fat provides long-term energy and helps store energy for future use.
- **Hormonal balance:** Fats are involved in the production of hormones, which regulate various bodily functions, including metabolism and reproduction.
- **Cell health:** Fat is a key component of cell membranes, supporting cell function and integrity.
- **Vitamin absorption:** Fat helps the body absorb fat-soluble vitamins (A, D, E, K) that support vision, bone health, immune function, and skin health.

Types of Fats:

a. Unsaturated Fats (healthy fats):

- **Monounsaturated fats:** Olive oil, avocados, nuts, seeds.
- **Polyunsaturated fats:** Fatty fish (salmon, mackerel), flaxseeds, walnuts.

b. **Saturated Fats:** Found in animal products (butter, cheese, fatty meats) and some plant oils (coconut oil, palm oil). It's best to consume these in moderation.

c. **Trans Fats:** Found in partially hydrogenated oils in processed foods (margarine, baked goods). These should be avoided, as they are linked to heart disease.

How Much Fat Do You Need?

- **General guideline:** Fat should make up about 20–35% of your total daily calories.
- **For weight loss or muscle building:** You can focus on healthy fats to maintain energy levels and promote fat loss.

How to Balance Macronutrients for Weight Loss

While all three macronutrients—protein, carbohydrates, and fats—are essential, the balance between them plays a key role in achieving your weight loss or health goals.

Recommended Macronutrient Ratio:

- **Protein:** 25-35% of your total daily calories (important for muscle repair and satiety).
- **Carbohydrates:** 40-50% of your total daily calories (focus on whole grains and vegetables for sustained energy).
- **Fats:** 25-35% of your total daily calories (prioritize healthy fats like those found in nuts, seeds, and fish).

Sample Macronutrient Breakdown (for a 2,000-calorie diet):

- **Protein:** 125–175 grams (500–700 calories)
- **Carbohydrates:** 200–250 grams (800–1,000 calories)
- **Fats:** 55–77 grams (500–700 calories)

CONCLUSION

The Pink Salt Trick Diet is a comprehensive approach to improving your overall health, supporting weight loss, and optimizing your metabolism. By incorporating Himalayan pink salt into your meals, you're not just enhancing flavor—you're benefiting from a rich source of essential minerals that help balance electrolytes, promote hydration, and support detoxification. However, it's important to remember that while pink salt can complement your health goals, it's just one part of a larger lifestyle that includes balanced eating, regular physical activity, and mindful habits.

As you continue your journey with the Pink Salt Trick Diet, focus on making sustainable changes that work for your body and lifestyle. Remember that consistency is key to achieving long-term success, and small, positive adjustments over time can lead to significant improvements in your health, energy, and well-being.

Key Takeaways:

1. **Balance is crucial:** Embrace the balance of protein, carbohydrates, and healthy fats in your diet. Moderation is key, especially when using pink salt.
2. **Hydration is essential:** Pink salt can enhance hydration, but drinking plenty of water should be a part of your daily routine.
3. **Patience and consistency:** Sustainable health improvements take time. Focus on building healthy habits that you can maintain long-term.
4. **Celebrate non-scale victories:** Progress is not just about weight loss—improvements in energy, digestion, and mood are just as important!
5. **Adjust as needed:** Be flexible and adapt the diet to your lifestyle as you move forward. If you miss a day or face challenges, get back on track without guilt.

Ultimately, the Pink Salt Trick Diet is about creating lasting changes that improve your quality of life. By focusing on whole, nutrient-dense foods, staying hydrated, and practicing portion control, you can achieve a healthier, more energized version of yourself.

Keep exploring new recipes, adjusting your routine, and making choices that support your goals. Stay committed to your wellness journey, and remember—it's about progress, not perfection.

FREE GIFT

SCAN THE QR CODE TO GET

YOUR FREE E-BOOK GIFT

DIVE INTO QUICK AND EASY RECIPES THAT ARE SURE TO INSPIRE YOUR CULINARY JOURNEY!

🙏 ACKNOWLEDGEMENTS

I would like to express my heartfelt gratitude to everyone who has supported and inspired me throughout the creation of **The Pink Salt Trick Diet for Weight Loss**. This book would not have been possible without the guidance, encouragement, and contributions of many individuals.

First and foremost, I would like to thank my family and friends for their unwavering support and belief in my vision. Their patience, understanding, and encouragement were crucial as I embarked on this journey.

A special thank you to the **health professionals**, **nutritionists**, and **dietitians** whose research and expertise have shaped the principles behind this book. Their guidance has been invaluable in ensuring the accuracy and effectiveness of the **Pink Salt Trick Diet.**

To my fellow wellness enthusiasts and the vibrant **online health community**—your feedback, shared experiences, and positive energy helped refine the content of this book. You've proven time and time again how important it is to come together and support one another on the path to better health.

I also want to acknowledge the **creators of the Pink Salt Trick Diet** and those who have shared their stories and results. Their experiences and successes have fueled my passion to share this diet with others who seek balance, wellness, and vitality.

Finally, a big thank you to **you, the reader**. It is your commitment to your health and your willingness to try new approaches that make this journey worthwhile. I hope this book becomes a helpful tool in your wellness journey, and I am excited to be part of your transformation.

Thank you to all who contributed to the creation of this book, and to those who are now embarking on this new chapter in their health journey.

RECIPE INDEX

A

Almond Butter Pink Salt Smoothie 51

Almond-Coconut Balls with a Pink Salt Twist 80

Asian Slaw with Pink Salt Sesame Dressing 62

Avocado Salsa with Pink Salt 76

Avocado Toast with Pink Salt & Chili Flakes 49

B

Baked Falafel with Pink Salt & Tahini Sauce 61

Baked Pink Salted Cod with Citrus Zest 67

Blueberry Protein Shake with Pink Salt 54

Breakfast Quinoa Bowl with Banana and Pink Salt 53

C

Chia Pudding with Pink Salted Mango 51

Chickpea Salad with Cucumber, Dill & Pink Salt 59

Cinnamon-Spiced Apple Bake with Pink Salt 54

D

Detox Smoothie with Cucumber, Mint & Pink Salt 78

F

Frozen Banana Bites with Pink Salt & Cocoa 82

G

Gluten-Free Breakfast Muffins with a Pink Salt Twist 55

Greek Yogurt Parfait with Pink Salted Granola 50

Green Smoothie with Lemon & Pink Salt 81

Grilled Chicken Salad with Pink Salt Citrus Dressing 58

Grilled Eggplant with Pink Salt Herb Drizzle 69

H

Herbed Basmati Rice with Pink Salt 70

L

Lemon Garlic Salmon with Pink Salt 66

Lentil Soup with Pink Salt and Thyme 60

M

Moroccan Chickpea Stew with Pink Salt 72

Mushroom and Pink Salt Risotto 63

O

Overnight Oats with Himalayan Sea Salt & Figs 52

P

Pink Salt & Turmeric Coconut Milk 55

Pink Salt Chicken Stir-Fry with Veggies 66

Pink Salt Chili Lime Chicken Skewers 71

Pink Salt Dark Chocolate Almond Bites 75

Pink Salt Edamame Pods 76

Pink Salt Marinated Grilled Tofu Bowl 62

Pink Salt Morning Detox Water 49

Pink Salt Nut & Seed Trail Mix 77

Pink Salt Sweet Potato Chips 75

Pink Salt Tuna Lettuce Wraps 58

Pink Salt Veggie Omelette 50

Pink Salt Watermelon & Mint Salad 78

Pink Salted Kale and Avocado Rice Bowl 61

Protein Bars with Pink Salt & Cranberries 79

Protein Pancakes with Pink Salted Berries 52

R

Roasted Seaweed Snack with Pink Salt 81

Roasted Turkey Meatballs with Pink Salt 68

Roasted Veggie & Quinoa Bowl with Pink Salt 59

S

Sautéed Spinach & Mushrooms with Pink Salt 69

Spiced Carrot Hummus with Pink Salt 77

Spicy Pink Salt Roasted Chickpeas 79

Stir-Fried Tofu and Broccoli in Pink Salt Sauce 68

Strawberry Coconut Shake with Pink Salt 80

Stuffed Bell Peppers with Pink Salt Quinoa Mix 64

Stuffed Zucchini Boats with Pink Salt 71

T

Teriyaki Glazed Tempeh with Pink Salt 73

Thai-Inspired Pink Salt Coconut Soup 72

Tofu Scramble with Pink Salt 53

Turmeric Chicken and Pink Salt Couscous 63

V

Vegan Cauliflower & Chickpea Curry 67

Z

Zesty Pink Salt Shrimp Stir-Fry 60

Zucchini Hash with Poached Egg and Pink Salt 56

Zucchini Noodles with Pink Salt Tomato Sauce 70

Notes

Printed in Dunstable, United Kingdom